YOGA ANATOMY

SECOND EDITION

Leslie Kaminoff

Amy Matthews

Illustrated by
Sharon Ellis

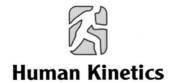

Human Kinetics

Library of Congress Cataloging-in-Publication Data

Kaminoff, Leslie, 1958-
  Yoga anatomy / Leslie Kaminoff, Amy Matthews ; Illustrated by Sharon
Ellis. -- 2nd ed.
    p. cm.
  Includes bibliographical references and indexes.
  ISBN-13: 978-1-4504-0024-4 (soft cover)
  ISBN-10: 1-4504-0024-8 (soft cover)
  1. Hatha yoga. 2. Human anatomy. I. Matthews, Amy. II. Title.
  RA781.7.K356 2011
  613.7'046--dc23

                        2011027333

ISBN-10: 1-4504-0024-8 (print)
ISBN-13: 978-1-4504-0024-4 (print)

This publication is written and published to provide accurate and authoritative information relevant to the subject matter presented. It is published and sold with the understanding that the author and publisher are not engaged in rendering legal, medical, or other professional services by reason of their authorship or publication of this work. If medical or other expert assistance is required, the services of a competent professional person should be sought.

The web addresses cited in this text were current as of August 2011, unless otherwise noted.

Managing Editor: Laura Podeschi; **Assistant Editors:** Claire Marty and Tyler Wolpert; **Copyeditor:** Joanna Hatzopoulos Portman; **Graphic Designer:** Joe Buck; **Graphic Artist:** Tara Welsch; **Original Cover Designer and Photographer (for illustration references):** Lydia Mann; **Photo Production Manager:** Jason Allen; **Art Manager:** Kelly Hendren; **Associate Art Manager:** Alan L. Wilborn; **Illustrations (cover and interior):** Sharon Ellis; **Printer:** Versa Press

Human Kinetics books are available at special discounts for bulk purchase. Special editions or book excerpts can also be created to specification. For details, contact the Special Sales Manager at Human Kinetics.

Printed in the United States of America   30 29 28 27

The paper in this book is certified under a sustainable forestry program.

Human Kinetics
P.O. Box 5076
Champaign, IL 61825-5076
Website: www.HumanKinetics.com

In the United States, email info@hkusa.com or call 800-747-4457.
In Canada, email info@hkcanada.com.
In the United Kingdom/Europe, email hk@hkeurope.com.

For information about Human Kinetics' coverage in other areas of the world, please visit our website: **www.HumanKinetics.com**

Tell us what you think!
Human Kinetics would love to hear what we can do to improve the customer experience. Use this QR code to take our brief survey.

To my teacher, T.K.V. Desikachar, I offer this book in gratitude for his unwavering insistence that I find my own truth. My greatest hope is that this work can justify his confidence in me.

And to my philosophy teacher, Ron Pisaturo—the lessons will never end.

—Leslie Kaminoff

In gratitude to all the students and teachers who have gone before—especially Philip, my student, teacher, and friend.

—Amy Matthews

CONTENTS

PREFACE

I am pleased to write this preface to an expanded, updated, and improved version of *Yoga Anatomy*. Most important, this new edition accurately reflects the true coauthorship of my collaborator and friend, Amy Matthews. In the first edition, I acknowledged working with Amy as one of the richest and most rewarding professional relationships I've ever had. At this point, a few years later in our collaboration, I remove the qualifier *one of*. When Amy and I work together, it is as if our complementary, individual knowledge and perspectives are specialized hemispheres that come together to act as a kind of superbrain. It is a truly joyous experience to work with someone who makes me exponentially smarter than when I'm alone. When we add the talent of Sharon Ellis, our extraordinary illustrator, as well as the support of our creative team at The Breathing Project, it makes for a potent mix.

Following the release of *Yoga Anatomy* in the summer of 2007, its success took everyone by surprise. As of this writing it has been translated into 19 languages, over 300,000 copies are in print, and it remains among the top-selling yoga books in the United States. We have received tremendous positive feedback from readers, many of whom are educators who now include *Yoga Anatomy* as a required text in their yoga teacher training courses. Practitioners as diverse as orthopedists, chiropractors, physical therapists, fitness trainers, and Pilates and Gyrotonic instructors are making good use of the book as well.

Some of the best feedback I've received revolves around the first two chapters centered on breath and spine. My intention in these chapters was to provide information I wish had been available to me 25 years ago when I was trying to figure out the anatomical basis of my teacher's distinctive approach to breathing in asana practice. I am especially pleased at how well received this information has been and am happy that this second edition provides the opportunity to add more illustrations, an expanded discussion of intrinsic equilibrium, the bandhas, and a brief history of the spine, deleted from the first edition due to space constraints.

Amy and I have also received critical feedback from readers, colleagues, and respected professionals in a variety of fields. The process of responding to this feedback has resulted in numerous improvements, the most significant of which are two new chapters by Amy on the skeletal system and the muscular system. These chapters feature a unique combination of sophistication and simplicity. The addition of these chapters makes *Yoga Anatomy* a more useful book that allows readers to better understand the specific anatomical terms used in the asana sections, especially joint actions and muscle actions.

Chapter 5 is a new jointly written chapter offering our analysis of the asanas and our approach to choosing what to analyze. You should read this chapter before reading any of the entries for the specific asanas, because it explains our unconventional and sometimes controversial perspectives on classification, breathing, and joint and muscle actions.

Amy has completely reviewed and revised the asana sections. She has eliminated arbitrary or confusing classifications, terms, and concepts and added information to clarify muscle actions and improve the overall consistency of presentation. Lydia Mann provided assistance in design by organizing the revised data as tables to offer ease of comprehension. Other improvements include additional asana variations and new indexes for illustrations of specific joints and muscles as well as corrections and relabeling of illustrations throughout.

Amy and I are confident that this new edition of *Yoga Anatomy* will continue to be a valuable resource for practitioners and teachers of yoga and all other forms of healthy movement. We hope you enjoy using it as much as we enjoyed putting it together. Please continue to let us know about your experiences in using the book.

Leslie Kaminoff
New York City
September 2011

ACKNOWLEDGMENTS

First and foremost, I express my gratitude to my family: Uma, Sasha, Jai, and Shaun. Their patience, understanding, love, and support have carried me through the lengthy process of conceiving, writing, editing, and revising this book. I wish also to thank my father and mother for supporting their son's unconventional interests and career for the past five decades. Allowing a child to find his own path in life is perhaps the greatest gift that a parent can give.

This has been a truly collaborative project that would never have happened without the ongoing support of a talented and dedicated team. Lydia Mann, whose most accurate title would be project and author wrangler, is a gifted designer, artist, and friend who guided me through every phase of this project: organizing, clarifying, and editing the structure of the book; shooting the majority of the photographs (including the author photos); and designing the covers. Without Lydia's partnership, this book would still be lingering somewhere in the space between my head and my hard drive.

Sharon Ellis has proven to be a skilled, perceptive, and flexible medical illustrator. When I first recruited her into this project after admiring her work online, she had no familiarity with yoga, but before long, she was slinging the Sanskrit terms and feeling her way through the postures like a seasoned yogi.

This book would never have existed had it not been originally conceived by the team at Human Kinetics. Martin Barnard's research led him to offer me the project. Leigh Keylock, Laura Podeschi, and Jason Muzinic's editorial guidance and encouragement kept the project on track. I can't thank them enough for their support and patience—mostly for their patience.

A very special thank-you goes to my literary agent and good friend, Bob Tabian, who has been a steady voice of reason and experience. He's the first person who saw me as an author, and he never lost faith that I could actually be one.

For education, inspiration, and coaching along the way, I thank Swami Vishnu Devananda, Lynda Huey, Leroy Perry Jr., Jack Scott, Larry Payne, Craig Nelson, Gary Kraftsow, Yan Dhyansky, Steve Schram, William LaSassier, David Gorman, Bonnie Bainbridge Cohen, Len Easter, Gil Hedley, and Tom Myers. I also thank all my students and clients past and present for being my most consistent and challenging teachers.

A big thank-you goes to all the models who posed for our images: Amy Matthews, Alana Kornfeld, Janet Aschkenasy, Mariko Hirakawa (our cover model), Steve Rooney (who also donated the studio at International Center of Photography for a major shoot), Eden Kellner, Elizabeth Luckett, Derek Newman, Carl Horowitz, J. Brown, Jyothi Larson, Nadiya Nottingham, Richard Freeman, Arjuna (Ronald Steiner), Eddie Stern, Shaun Kaminoff, and Uma McNeill. Thanks also to the Krishnamacharya Yoga Mandiram for permission to use the iconic photos of T. Krishnamacharya as reference for the Mahamudra and Mulabandhasana drawings.

Invaluable support for this project was provided by Jen Harris, Edya Kalev, Alana Kramer, Leandro Willaro, Rudi Bach, Jenna O'Brien, Sarah Barnaby, and all the teachers, staff, students, and supporters of The Breathing Project.

Leslie Kaminoff

I begin by thanking Leslie for his generosity of spirit. Since he initially invited me to be a part of The Breathing Project in 2003, he has unfailingly supported my approach to teaching, recommended my classes and workshops to his students, and invited me to be a part of the creation of this book.

Little did I know what would come when he approached me to help with a cool idea he had about a book on yoga anatomy! In the process of creating the initial book and this second edition, he and I have had many conversations in which we questioned and challenged and elaborated on each other's ideas in a way that has polished and refined what we both have to offer.

For me to be the educator that I now am, I first thank my family. My parents both encouraged me to question and to understand for myself. My father was always willing to explain something to me, and my mother encouraged me to go look it up and figure it out. From them, I learned I could do my own research and form my own ideas . . . and no detail was too small to consider!

Thanks to all the teachers who encouraged my curiosity and passion for understanding things: Alison West, for cultivating a spirit of exploration and inquiry in her yoga classes; Mark Whitwell, for constantly reminding me of what I already know about why I am a teacher; Irene Dowd, for her enthusiasm and precision; Gil Hedley, for his willingness to not know and still dive in and learn; and Bonnie Bainbridge Cohen, who models the passion and compassion for herself and her students that lets her be such a gift as a teacher.

Several people have been instrumental in the process of creating the new material in the second edition. Tremendous thanks to Chloe Chung Misner for reading every draft of the new chapters and reminding me to be in my bones. Michelle Gay also kept wanting to know more and asked incredibly useful questions. The students at The Breathing Project have continued to inspire me as a teacher. The staff at The Breathing Project, especially Alana, Edya, Alyson, and Alicia, have done an incredible job of keeping the space running when Leslie and I have been consumed by this process.

Sarah Barnaby has been an invaluable colleague in helping me refine the asana material in the second edition, brainstorming ideas for images, and in general reminding me of what I mean to say. She also prepared the material for the indexes and proofread at every step of the way.

I am grateful to all the people who helped me in the process of working on this book: my dearest friends Michelle and Aynsley; Karen, whose support sustained me in creating the first edition; our BMC summer kitchen table circle, Wendy, Elizabeth, and Tarina; Kidney and all the people I told to stop asking about the book; and the BMC students who welcomed me and gave me feedback, especially Moonshadow, Raven-Light, Michael, Rosemary, and Jesse. And a loving thank-you to Sarah, who continues to inspire me to be more expansive and creative about my life and my teaching than I had ever thought possible.

Amy Matthews

INTRODUCTION

This book is by no means an exhaustive study of human anatomy or the vast science of yoga. No single book could be. Both fields contain a potentially infinite number of details, both macro- and microscopic, all of which are endlessly fascinating and potentially useful depending on your interests. Our intention is to present the details of anatomy that are of most value to people involved in yoga whether as students or as teachers.

THE TRUE SELF IS AN EMBODIED SELF

Yoga speaks of getting at something deep inside of us—the true self. The goal of this quest is often stated in mystical terms, implying that our true selves exist on some nonmaterial plane. This book takes the opposing stand that in order to go deeply inside ourselves, we must journey within our physical bodies. Once there, we will not only understand our anatomy but also directly experience the reality that gives rise to the core concepts of yoga. This is a truly embodied experience of spirituality. We make a clear distinction between mystical (the claim to the perception of a supernatural reality experienced by some extrasensory means) and spiritual (from the Latin *spiritus,* meaning breath, the animating, sensitive, or vital principle of the individual).

The reason for this mutually illuminating relationship between yoga and anatomy is simple: The deepest principles of yoga are based on a subtle and profound appreciation of how the human system is constructed. The subject of yoga is the self, and the self is an attribute of a physical body.

PRACTICE, DISCERNMENT, AND SURRENDER

The ancient teachings we've inherited were developed through the enlightened observation of life in all its forms and expressions. The skillful observation of humans gave rise to the possibility of yoga practice (kriya yoga) classically formulated by Patañjali and restated by Reinhold Niebuhr in his famous serenity prayer.[1] Within this practice we orient our attitudes toward the discernment (swadhyaya) to distinguish the things we can change (tapah) from the things we cannot change (isvara pranidhana).

Isn't this a prime motivation to study anatomy in the context of yoga? We want to know what's inside of us so we can understand why some things are relatively easy to change and others seem so difficult. How much energy should we devote to working through our own resistance? When should we work on surrendering to something that's not likely to change? Both require effort. Surrender is an act of will. These are never-ending questions with answers that seem to change every day—precisely why we must never stop posing them.

A little anatomical knowledge goes a long way in this pursuit, especially when we include the subject of breathing in our inquiry. What makes the breath such a potent teacher of yoga? Breathing has the dual nature of being both voluntary and autonomic, which is why the breath illuminates the eternal inquiry about what we can control or change and what we cannot. We all face this personal yet universal inquiry at some point if we desire to evolve.

---

[1] Karl Paul Reinhold Niebuhr (1892–1971), American theologian: "Grant to us the serenity of mind to accept that which cannot be changed, courage to change that which can be changed, and wisdom to know the one from the other."

WELCOME TO MY LABORATORY

The context that yoga provides for the study of anatomy is rooted in the exploration of how our life force expresses itself through the movements of the body, breath, and mind. The ancient metaphorical language of yoga has arisen from anatomical experimentations by millions of seekers over thousands of years. All these seekers shared a common laboratory—their human bodies. This book provides a guided tour of this lab, with descriptions on function of the equipment and the basic procedures that yield insights. Rather than offer a manual for the practice of a particular system of yoga, we offer a solid grounding in the principles of the physical practice of all systems of yoga.

Because yoga practice emphasizes the relationship of the breath and the spine, we pay particular attention to those systems. By viewing all other body structures in light of their relationship to the breath and spine, yoga becomes the integrating principle for the study of anatomy. Additionally, we honor the yogic perspective of dynamic interconnectedness by avoiding reductionist analysis of the poses and prescriptive listings of their benefits.

ALL WE NEED IS ALREADY PRESENT

The ancient yogis held the view that we actually have three bodies: physical, astral, and causal. From this perspective, yoga anatomy is the study of the subtle currents of energy that move through the layers, or sheaths, of those three bodies. The purpose of this work is to neither support nor refute this view. We simply offer the perspective that if you are reading this book, you have a mind and a body that are currently inhaling and exhaling in a gravitational field. Therefore, you can benefit immensely from a process that enables you to think more clearly, breathe more effortlessly, and move more efficiently. This is, in fact, our starting point and definition of yoga practice: the integration of mind, breath, and body.

Another ancient principle tells us that the main task of yoga practice is the removal of obstacles that impede the natural functioning of our systems. This sounds simple enough but runs counter to a common feeling that our problems are due to something that's lacking, or missing. What yoga can teach us is that everything essential we need for our health and happiness is already present in our systems. We merely need to identify and resolve some of the obstacles that obstruct those natural forces from operating, "like a farmer who cuts a dam to allow water to flow into the field where it is needed."[2] This is great news for anyone regardless of age, infirmity, or inflexibility; if there is breath and mind, then there can be yoga.

FROM THE CRADLE TO GRAVITY

Rather than see the body's musculature as a system of pulleys and fulcrums that needs to function as a counterforce to gravity, we see the body as a dynamically coupled series of spiraling tubes, channels, and chambers that support themselves from the inside.

Some of this support operates independently of the action of the musculature and its metabolic demands. We call this principle intrinsic equilibrium, and its workings are observable in the way the spine, rib cage, and pelvis are knit together under mechanical tension. The cavities contained by those structures exhibit a pressure differential that makes our organ systems gravitate upward toward the body's region of lowest pressure in the rib cage.

Why does it take practice to learn how to tap into these deep sources of internal support? Habitual tension accumulates over a lifetime of operating our muscular pulleys and

---

[2] From *Yoga Sutras* by Patañjali, chapter 4, sutra 3, in *The Heart of Yoga: Developing Personal Practice* by T.K.V. Desikachar (Inner Traditions International, 1995).

fulcrums against the constant pull of gravity, and the constant modulation of our breathing patterns is invoked as a way of regulating our internal emotional landscape. These postural and breath habits operate mostly unconsciously unless some intentional change (tapah) is introduced into the system by a practice like yoga. This is why we often refer to yoga as a controlled stress experience.

In this context, the practice of asana becomes a systematic exploration of unobstructing the deeper self-supporting forces of breath and posture. We offer suggestions for alignment, breathing, and awareness that can help in this exploration in the asana sections of this book.

Rather than view asana practice as a way of *imposing* order on the human system, we encourage you to use the poses as a way of *uncovering* the intrinsic order that nature put there. This doesn't mean we ignore issues of alignment, placement, and sequencing. We simply maintain that achieving proper alignment is a means to a greater end, not an end in itself. We don't live to do yoga; we do yoga so that we may *live*—more easily, joyously, and gracefully.

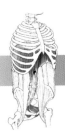

CHAPTER 1

DYNAMICS OF BREATHING

This chapter explores breath anatomy from a yogic perspective, using the cell as a starting point. This most basic unit of life can teach us an enormous amount about yoga. In fact, we can derive the most essential yogic concepts from observing the cell's form and function. Furthermore, when we understand the basics of a single cell, we can understand the basics of anything made out of cells, such as the human body.

YOGA LESSONS FROM A CELL

Cells are the fundamental building blocks of life, from single-celled plants to multitrillion-celled animals. The human body, which is made up of roughly 100 trillion cells, begins as two newly created cells.

A cell consists of three parts: the cell membrane, the nucleus, and the cytoplasm. The membrane separates a cell's internal environment, which consists of the cytoplasm and nucleus, from its external environment, which contains the nutrients that the cell requires.

After nutrients have penetrated the membrane, they are metabolized and turned into energy that fuels a cell's life functions. An unavoidable by-product of all metabolic activity is waste, which must get back out through the same membrane. Any impairment to a cell's ability to let nutrients in or let waste out results in death by starvation or toxicity. The yogic concepts that relate to this functional activity of the cell are prana and apana. The concepts that relate to the structural properties of the membrane that support that function are sthira and sukha.

Prana and Apana

The Sanskrit term *prana* is derived from *pra-*, a prefix meaning before, and *an*, a verb meaning to breathe, to blow, and to live. *Prana* refers to what nourishes a living thing, but it has also come to mean the action that brings the nourishment in. Within this chapter, the term will refer to the functional life processes of a single entity. When capitalized, *Prana* is a more universal term that can be used to designate the manifestation of all creative life force.

All living systems require a balance of forces, and the yogic concept that complements prana is *apana*, which is derived from *apa*, meaning away, off, or down. Apana refers to the waste that's being eliminated as well as the action of elimination. These two fundamental yogic terms—*prana* and *apana*—encompass the essential functions of life on every level, from cell to organism.

Sthira and Sukha

If prana and apana are expressions of function, what of the structural conditions that have to exist in a cell in order for nutrition to enter and waste to exit? This is the function of the membrane—a structure that must be just permeable enough to allow material to pass in and out (see figure 1.1, page 2). If the membrane is too permeable, the cell loses integrity, causing it to either explode from pressures within or implode from pressures without.

In a cell, as in all living things, the principle that balances permeability is stability. The yogic terms that reflect these polarities are *sthira* and *sukha*. In Sanskrit, *sthira* can mean firm, hard, solid, compact, strong, unfluctuating, durable, lasting, or permanent. *Sukha* is composed of two roots: *su* meaning good and *kha* meaning space. It means easy, pleasant, agreeable, gentle, and mild. It also refers to a state of well-being, free of obstacles.

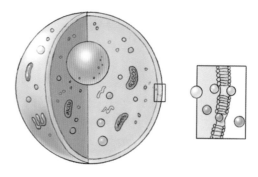

All successful living things must balance containment and permeability, rigidity and plasticity, persistence and adaptability, and space and boundaries. This is how life avoids destruction through starvation or toxicity and through implosion or explosion.

Figure 1.1   The cell's membrane must balance containment (stability) with permeability.

Successful man-made structures also exhibit a balance of sthira and sukha. For example, a suspension bridge is flexible enough to survive wind and earthquakes, but stable enough to support its load-bearing surfaces. This image also invokes the principles of tension and compression, which are discussed in chapter 2.

Sukha also means having a good axle hole, implying a space at the center that allows function. Like a wheel, a person needs to have good space at his or her center, or functional connections become impossible.

Human Pathways of Prana and Apana: Nutrition In, Waste Out

The body's pathways for nutrients and waste are not as simple as those of a cell, but not so complex that we can't easily describe them in terms of prana and apana.

Figure 1.2 shows a simplified version of our nutritional and waste pathways. It shows how the human system is open at the top and at the bottom. We take in prana—solid and liquid nourishment—at the top of the system. These solids and liquids enter the alimentary canal, move through the digestive process, and, after a lot of twists and turns, move down and out as waste matter. This is the only way waste can go, because the exits are at the bottom. It is clear that the force of apana, when acting on solid and liquid waste, must move down to get out.

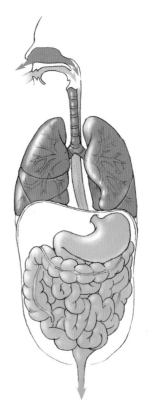

Figure 1.2   Solid and liquid nutrition (blue) enter at the top of the system and exit as waste at the bottom. Gaseous nutrition and waste (red) enter and exit at the top.

Prana also enters our bodies in gaseous form: the breath. Like solids and liquids, it enters at the top, where it remains above the diaphragm in the lungs (see figure 1.3), exchanging gases with the capillaries at the alveoli. The waste gas in the lungs needs to be expelled, but it gets out the same way it came in. The force of apana, when acting on respiratory waste gas, must move up to get out. Apana must be able to operate freely both upward and downward, depending on what type of waste it acts upon.

The ability to reverse apana's downward action is a basic and useful skill acquired through yoga practice, but not something most people are able to do without training. People are accustomed to pushing down to operate their apana. Many have learned that whenever something needs to be eliminated from the body, the body must squeeze in and push down. That is why, when most beginning students are asked to exhale completely, they activate their breathing muscles as if they are urinating or defecating.

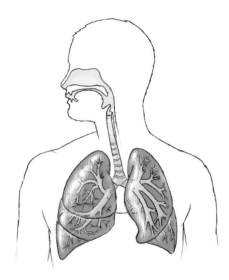

Figure 1.3 The pathway that air takes into and out of the body.

Sukha and Dukha

Prana and apana must have a healthy reciprocal relationship in the body; thus, the body's pathways must be clear of obstructing forces. In yogic terms, our breathing bodies must be in a state of *sukha*, translated literally as good space. Bad space is referred to as *dukha*, which is derived from *dus*, meaning bad, difficult, or hard, and *kha*, meaning space. It is generally translated as suffering, uneasy, uncomfortable, unpleasant, and difficult.

This model points to the fundamental methodology of all classical yoga practice, which seeks to uncover and resolve blockages or obstructions (kleshas[1]) to improve function. Essentially, when we make more good space our pranic forces flow freely and restore normal, healthy function.

The modern master of yoga therapy, T.K.V. Desikachar, has often said that yoga therapy is 90 percent waste removal.

Because exhalation is an action of removing waste from the system, another practical way of applying this insight is that if we take care of the exhalation, the inhalation takes care of itself. If we get rid of the unwanted, we make room for what is needed.

Being Born to Breath and Gravity

When a fetus is in utero, the mother does the breathing. Her lungs deliver oxygen to the uterus and placenta. From there it travels to the umbilical cord, which takes about half the oxygenated blood to the inferior vena cava while the other half enters the liver. The two sides of the heart are connected, bypassing the lungs, which remain dormant until the child is born. Needless to say, human fetal circulation is very different from ex-utero circulation.

---

[1] *Klestr* means that which causes pain or suffering.

Being born means being severed from the umbilical cord—the lifeline that has sustained the fetus for nine months. Suddenly, and for the first time, the infant needs to engage in actions that ensure continued survival. The very first of these actions declares physical and physiological independence. It is the first breath, and it is the most important and forceful inhalation a human will ever take.

The initial inflation of the lungs triggers enormous changes to the entire circulatory system, which has previously been geared toward receiving oxygenated blood from the placenta. That first breath causes a massive surge of blood into the lungs, the right and left sides of the heart to separate into two pumps, and the specialized vessels of fetal circulation to shut down, seal off, and become ligaments that support the abdominal organs.

That first inhalation must be so forceful because it needs to overcome the initial surface tension of the previously inactive lung tissue. The force required to overcome that tension is three or four times greater than that of a normal inhalation.[2]

Another radical reversal that occurs at the moment of birth is the sudden experience of body weight in space. Inside the womb, the fetus is in a cushioned, supportive, fluid-filled environment. Suddenly, the child's entire universe expands—the limbs and head can move freely, and the baby must be supported in gravity.

Because adults swaddle babies and move them around from place to place, stability and mobility may not seem to be so much of an issue early in life. In fact, infants begin to develop their posture immediately after taking their first breath, as soon as they begin to nurse. The complex, coordinated action of simultaneously breathing, sucking, and swallowing eventually provides them with the tonic strength to accomplish their first postural skill—supporting the weight of the head. This is no small feat for the infant, considering that an infant's head constitutes one fourth of its overall body length, compared to one eighth for an adult.

Head support involves the coordinated action of many muscles and, as with all weight-bearing skills, a balancing act between mobilization and stabilization. Postural development continues from the head downward until after about a year, when babies begin walking, culminating in the completion of the lumbar curve at about 10 years of age (see chapter 2).

Having a healthy life on Earth requires an integrated relationship between breath and posture, prana and apana, and sthira and sukha. If something goes wrong with one of these functions, by definition it will go wrong with the others. In this light, yoga practice can be viewed as a way of integrating the body's systems so we spend more time in a state of sukha than in dukha.

To summarize, from the moment of birth, humans are confronted by breath and gravity, two forces that were not present in utero. To thrive, we need to reconcile those forces as long as we draw breath on this planet.

BREATHING DEFINED: MOVEMENT IN TWO CAVITIES

Breathing is traditionally defined in medical texts as the process of taking air into and expelling it from the lungs. This process—the passage of air into and out of the lungs—is movement; specifically, it is movement in the body's cavities, which I will refer to as shape change. So, for the purposes of this exploration, here's our definition:

Breathing is the shape change of the body's cavities.

---

[2] The initial inflation of the lungs is assisted by the presence of surfactant, a substance that lowers the surface tension of the stiff, newborn lung tissue. Because surfactant is produced very late in intrauterine life, babies who are born prematurely (before 28 weeks of gestation) have a hard time breathing.

The simplified illustration of the human body in figure 1.4 shows that the torso consists of two cavities, thoracic and abdominal. These cavities share some properties, and they have important distinctions as well. Both contain vital organs: The thoracic cavity contains the heart and lungs, and the abdominal cavity contains the stomach, liver, gall bladder, spleen, pancreas, small and large intestines, kidneys, and bladder.

Both cavities open at one end to the external environment—the thoracic at the top, and the abdominal at the bottom. The cavities open to each other[3] by means of an important shared, dividing structure, the diaphragm. Another important shared property is that both cavities are bound posteriorly by the spine. The two cavities also share the quality of mobility—they change shape. This shape-changing ability is most relevant to breathing; without this movement, the body cannot breathe at all.

Although both the abdominal and thoracic cavities change shape, an important structural difference exists in how they do so.

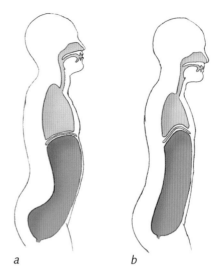

Figure 1.4 Breathing is thoracoabdominal shape change between *(a)* inhalation and *(b)* exhalation.

The Water Balloon and the Accordion

The abdominal cavity changes shape like a flexible, fluid-filled structure such as a water balloon. When you squeeze one end of a water balloon, the other end bulges (figure 1.5).

That is because water is noncompressible. Your hand's action only moves the fixed volume of water from one region of the flexible container to another. The same principle applies when the movements of breathing compress the abdominal cavity; a squeeze in one region produces a bulge in another. In the context of breathing, the abdominal cavity changes shape but not volume. In the context of life processes other than breathing, the abdominal cavity does change volume. When you drink a large volume of liquid or eat a big meal, the overall volume of the abdominal cavity increases as a result of expanded abdominal organs (stomach, intestines, and bladder). Any volume increase in the abdominal cavity produces a corresponding decrease in the volume of the thoracic cavity. That is why it is more difficult to breathe after a big meal, before a big bowel movement, or when pregnant.

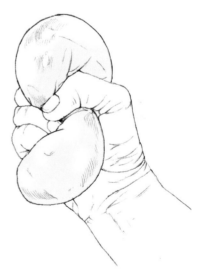

Figure 1.5 The water balloon changes shape but not volume.

---

[3] The three openings (hiati) in the diaphragm are for the arterial supply to the lower body (aortic hiatus), the venous return from the lower body to the heart (inferior vena cava) and the esophagus (esophageal hiatus). *Hiatus* is the Latin past participle of *hiare*—to stand open or yawn.

In contrast to the abdominal cavity, the thoracic cavity changes both shape and volume; it behaves as a flexible gas-filled container, similar to an accordion bellows. When you squeeze an accordion, you create a reduction in the volume of the bellows and air is forced out. When you pull the bellows open, its volume increases and air is pulled in (figure 1.6). This occurs because the accordion is compressible and expandable, as is air. The same is true of the thoracic cavity, which, unlike the abdominal cavity and its contents, can change its shape and volume in breathing.

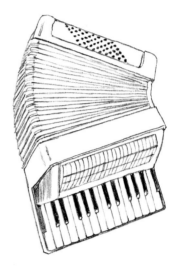

Let's now imagine the thoracic and abdominal cavities as an accordion stacked on top of a water balloon. This image gives a sense of the relationship of the two cavities in breathing; movement in one will necessarily result in movement in the other. Recall that during an inhalation (the shape change permitting air to be pushed into the lungs by the planet's atmospheric pressure), the thoracic cavity expands its volume. This pushes downward on the abdominal cavity, which changes shape as a result of the pressure from above.

Figure 1.6   The accordion changes shape and volume.

By defining breathing as shape change, it becomes very easy to understand what constitutes effective or obstructed breath—it is simply the ability or inability of the structures that define and surround the body's cavities to change shape.

The Universe Breathes Us

Volume and pressure are inversely related; when volume increases, pressure decreases, and when volume decreases, pressure increases. Because air always flows toward areas of lower pressure, increasing the volume inside the thoracic cavity will decrease pressure and cause air to flow into it. This is an inhalation.

It is important to note that in spite of how it feels when you inhale, you do not actually pull air into the body. On the contrary, air is pushed into the body by the atmospheric pressure (14.7 pounds per square inch, or 1.03 kg/cm^2) that always surrounds you. This means that the actual force that gets air into the lungs is outside of the body. The energy expended in breathing produces a shape change that lowers the pressure in the chest cavity and permits the air to be pushed into the body by the weight of the planet's atmosphere. In other words, you create the space, and the universe fills it.

During relaxed, quiet breathing such as while sleeping, an exhalation is a passive reversal of this process. The thoracic cavity and lung tissue—which have been stretched open during the inhalation—spring back to their initial volume, pushing the air out and returning them to their previous shapes. This is referred to as a *passive recoil*. Any reduction in the elasticity of these tissues results in a reduction of the body's ability to exhale passively, leading to a host of respiratory problems such as emphysema and pulmonary fibrosis, which greatly compromise the elasticity of the lung tissue.

In breathing patterns that involve active exhaling, such as blowing out candles, speaking, singing, and performing various yoga exercises, the musculature surrounding the two cavities contracts in such a way that the abdominal cavity is pushed upward into the thoracic cavity or the thoracic cavity is pushed downward onto the abdominal cavity, or any combination of the two.

Three-Dimensional Shape Changes of Breathing

Because the lungs occupy a three-dimensional space in the thoracic cavity, when this space changes shape to cause air movement, it changes shape three-dimensionally. Specifically, an inhalation involves the chest cavity increasing its volume from top to bottom, from side to side, and from front to back, and an exhalation involves a reduction of volume in those three dimensions (see figure 1.7).

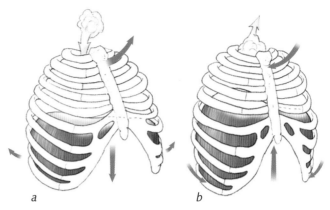

Figure 1.7   Three-dimensional thoracic shape changes of *(a)* inhalation and *(b)* exhalation.

Because thoracic shape change is inextricably linked to abdominal shape change, you can also say that the abdominal cavity also changes shape (not volume) in three dimensions—it can be squeezed from top to bottom, from side to side, or from front to back (see figure 1.8). In a living, breathing body, thoracic shape change cannot occur without abdominal shape change. That is why the condition of the abdominal region has such an influence on the quality of our breathing and why the quality of our breathing has a powerful effect on the health of our abdominal organs.

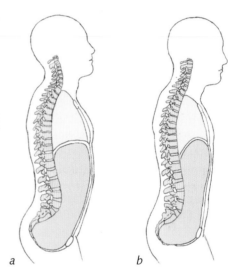

Figure 1.8   Changes in abdominal shape during breathing: *(a)* inhalation as spinal extension and *(b)* exhalation as spinal flexion.

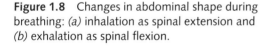

EXPANDED DEFINITION OF BREATHING

Based on the information we have so far, here's an expanded definition of breathing:

> *Breathing, the process of taking air into and expelling it from the lungs, is caused by a three-dimensional shape change in the thoracic and abdominal cavities.*

Defining breathing in this manner explains not only what it is but also how it is done. As a thought experiment, try this: Substitute the term *shape change* for the word *breathing* whenever discussing the breath. For example, "I just had a really good breath" really means "I just had a really good shape change." More important, "I'm having difficulty breathing" really means "I'm having trouble changing the shape of my cavities." This concept has profound therapeutic implications, because it tells us where to start looking for the root causes of breath and postural issues, and it can eventually lead us to examine the supporting, shape-changing structure that occupies the back of the body's two primary cavities—the spine, which is discussed in chapter 2.

A key observation that has been made in yogic teachings is that spinal movements are an intrinsic component of the shape-changing activity of the cavities (breathing). This is why such a huge component of yoga practice involves coordinating the movements of the spine with the process of inhaling and exhaling.

There's a reason why students are instructed to inhale during spinal extension and exhale during spinal flexion. Fundamentally, the spinal shape change of extension is an inhale and the spinal shape change of spinal flexion is an exhale.

THE DIAPHRAGM'S ROLE IN BREATHING

A single muscle, the diaphragm, is capable of producing—on its own—all of the three-dimensional movements of breath. This is why just about every anatomy book describes the diaphragm as the principal muscle of breathing. Let's add the diaphragm to our shape-change definition of breathing to begin our exploration of this remarkable muscle:

> The diaphragm is the principal muscle that causes three-dimensional shape change in the thoracic and abdominal cavities.

To understand how the diaphragm causes this shape change, it is important to examine its shape and location in the body, where it is attached and what is attached to it, its action, and its relationship to the other muscles of breathing.

Shape and Location

The deeply domed shape of the diaphragm has evoked many images. Two of the most common are a jellyfish and a parachute (figure 1.9). It is important to note that the diaphragm's shape is created by the organs it encloses and supports. Deprived of its relationship with those organs, its dome would collapse, much like a stocking cap without a head in it. It is also evident that the diaphragm has an asymmetrical double-dome shape; the right dome rises higher than the left. The liver pushes up from below the right dome, and the heart pushes down from above the left dome (see figure 1.10 on page 9).

The diaphragm divides the torso into the thoracic and abdominal cavities. It is the floor of the thoracic cavity and the roof of the abdominal cavity. Its structure extends through

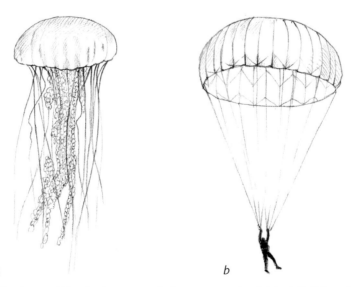

a   *b*

Figure 1.9 The shape of the diaphragm reminds many people of *(a)* a jellyfish or *(b)* a parachute.

a wide section of the body. The uppermost part reaches the space between the third and fourth ribs, and its lowest fibers attach to the front of the third and second lumbar vertebrae; nipple to navel is one way to describe it.

Muscular Attachments of the Diaphragm

Muscles attach at origin and insertion points. The determination of origin or insertion is dependent on two factors: structure and function.

- Structurally, the end of the muscle closest to the core of the body—the proximal end—is usually referred to as the origin. The distal end, the one that attaches more peripherally, is usually referred to as the insertion.

- Functionally, the end of the muscle that is more stable on contraction is referred to as the origin, and the more mobile end the insertion.

Although this seems to make sense—proximal structures are generally more stable than distal ones—this is only true some of the time, as is explored further in chapter 4. For example, a reversal of functional origins and insertions occurs when you have a mobile core and stable extremities while moving the body through space.

The muscle that moves space through the body—the diaphragm—possesses an unmistakably three-dimensional form and function, which makes its origin and insertion anything but cut and dried. To avoid confusion as we begin to examine the attachments of its muscular fibers, we simply refer to the diaphragm's lower attachments and upper attachments.

Lower Attachments

The lower edges of the diaphragm's fibers attach at four distinct regions. Traditional texts list only three regions: sternal, costal, and lumbar (see figure 1.10).

1. **Sternal**—The back of the xiphoid process at the bottom of the sternum

2. **Costal**—The inner costal cartilage surfaces of ribs 6 through 10

3. **Arcuate**—The arcuate ligament[4] that runs from rib 10's cartilage to the lumbar spine, attaching along the way to the floating ribs (11 and 12) and the transverse process and body of L1

4. **Lumbar**—The crura (Latin for legs) at the front of the lumbar spine, L3 on right and L2 on left

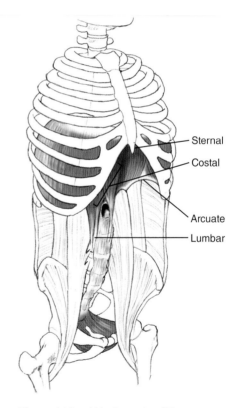

Sternal

Costal

Arcuate

Lumbar

Figure 1.10   Attachments of the diaphragm muscle.

---

[4] Traditional texts label each arc of the arcuate ligament individually. It is much clearer to think of it as a single, long ligament that attaches to the tips of the bony surfaces mentioned. In dissection, when the arcuate ligament is deprived of these attachments, it clearly stretches out into a single, straight ligament.

Upper Attachments

All the muscular fibers of the diaphragm rise upward in the body from their lower attachments. They eventually arrive at the flattened, horizontal top of the muscle, the central tendon, into which they blend. In essence, the diaphragm connects to itself—its own center, which is fibrous noncontractile tissue. The central tendon's vertical movements within the body are limited by its strong connection to the heart's fibrous pericardium, to which it is inextricably linked.

Traditional texts refer to the lower attachments as the muscle's origin, and the central tendon as the insertion. The following text offers our reevaluation of that assumption.

Challenging Traditional Labeling of Origin and Insertion

As we will see later in this chapter, there is much confusion among breathing teachers about the action of the diaphragm. Why is there so much confusion, and where did it begin? A major factor may be that the structural origin and insertion of the diaphragm have historically been mislabeled in anatomy texts. This has resulted in a functional confusion about which end of the muscle is stable and which is mobile when the diaphragm's fibers contract.

Assumptions About Structure   In terms of structure, traditional anatomy texts present the origin of the diaphragm as its lower attachments, and the central tendon is labeled as its insertion. Upon closer scrutiny, this categorization breaks down.

Let's see how true this is for the location of your diaphragm's lower attachments (see figure 1.10 on page 9). If you place your fingertips at the base of your sternum, you can usually touch the tip of your xiphoid process. You can then sweep your fingers around the edges of your costal cartilage, and from there around your back to the region of the floating ribs, and then to the top of your lumbar spine.

At every point of contact you just traced on your body, your fingertips were as little as 1/4 inch (0.6 cm) and no more than one 1 inch (2.5 cm) away from the sternal, costal, arcuate, or lumbar attachments of your diaphragm. Your fingers were on the surface of your body, not near its core, and neither were the attachments you just traced.

Now, let's see if you can trace your diaphragm's upper attachments. Can you get your fingertips close to your central tendon? Not really, because it is at the core of the body. In fact, your heart is anchored to it. Describing this structure as *central* is apt, which is why using a term that is usually reserved for distal structures (insertion) is all the more confusing.

Lower Fibers   The lower muscular fibers of the diaphragm attach to flexible cartilage and ligament. The bottom of the xiphoid process is mostly cartilage. The costal cartilage is springy and flexible and has many joints that attach it to the ribs, which are among the more than 100 joints that make up the rib cage articulations. The arcuate ligament is a long, ropy band that attaches to the tips of the floating ribs. The front surface of the lumbar spine is covered with the anterior longitudinal ligament, which is anchored to the anterior surfaces of the cartilaginous intervertebral discs as well as the anterior surfaces of the lumbar vertebrae.

Assuming that the rib cage is allowed to move freely, we can make a strong case that these lower attachments of the diaphragm have considerable potential for movement. Even the crura have this potential in situations involving lumbar motion and the action of the psoas muscles, which share common attachments in the upper lumbar region.

Upper Fibers   The center of the diaphragm and the heart have never been apart. The tissue that will become the central tendon actually originates outside of the thoracic cavity in our embryonic development. At this early stage, it is called the transverse septum, and it lies adjacent to the primordial heart tissue. With the inward folding of the embryo's structure in the fourth week in utero, the heart and transverse septum move together into the thoracic cavity. Once the transverse septum is in this location, the muscular tissue of the diaphragm grows toward it from the interior surface of the abdominal wall. Thus, the association of the central tendon with the heart is the original manifestation of the diaphragm, and further justifies labeling it as its origin.

Because of its firm anchorage to the heart, the tough, fibrous tissue of the central tendon has limited ability to move vertically within the thoracic cavity (between 1/2 to 1 inch). Therefore, the upper muscular attachments of the diaphragm closest to the central tendon have little movement potential. However, the muscular domes that rise up on either side of the central tendon do have the ability to strongly push downward on the abdominal viscera, and this (not the downward movement of the central tendon itself) mostly accounts for the bulging of the upper abdomen commonly referred to as a belly breath.

Conclusions   For all the reasons just mentioned, we have concluded that traditional texts reverse the structural labeling of origin and insertion of the diaphragm by describing distal structures (lower attachments) as origin and proximal structures (upper attachments) as insertion. This structural confusion leads to a functional confusion because of the assumption that muscular insertions are mobile and muscular origins are stable. We will explore this shortly.

Organic Relations

Studying the diaphragm's origin and insertion allows us to understand what structures it is attached to. But unlike other muscles, the diaphragm has a lot of structures attached to it. This is what is meant by the term *organic relations*.

As the prime mover of the thoracic and abdominal cavities, the diaphragm is a place of anchorage for the connective tissue that surrounds the thoracic and abdominal organs. The names of these important structures are easily remembered as the three Ps:

- Pleura, which surrounds the lungs
- Pericardium, which surrounds the heart
- Peritoneum, which surrounds the abdominal organs

It should be clear that the shape-changing activity of these cavities has a profound effect on the movements of the organs they contain. The diaphragm is a fundamental source of these movements, but the viscera are also a source of resistance and stabilization for the diaphragm. This reciprocal relationship illuminates why the coordinated movements of breath and body promoted by yoga practice can lead to such dramatic improvements in the overall health and functioning of all the body's systems.

Action of the Diaphragm

It is important to remember that the muscular fibers of the diaphragm are oriented primarily along the vertical (up–down) axis of the body (see figure 1.11).

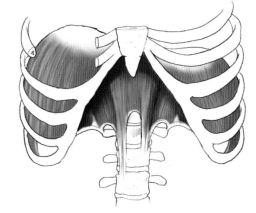

Figure 1.11   The muscular fibers of the diaphragm all run vertically from their lower attachments to the central tendon.

As with all muscles, the contracting fibers of the diaphragm pull their two ends (the central tendon and the base of the rib cage) toward each other. This action is the fundamental cause of the three-dimensional thoracoabdominal shape changes of breathing.

Because the diaphragm has multidimensional action, the type of movement it produces depends on which region of its attachment is stable and which is mobile.

To illustrate this with a more visible movement, the psoas major muscle creates hip flexion either by moving the leg toward the front of the spine, as in standing on one leg and flexing the opposite hip, or by moving the front of the spine toward the leg, as in sit-ups with the legs braced. In both cases, the psoas major is contracting and flexing the hip joint. What differs is which end of the muscle is stable and which is mobile. Needless to say, a stable torso and moving leg look very different from a moving torso and a stable leg.

Variety of Diaphragmatic Breaths

Just as you can think of the psoas major as either a leg mover or a trunk mover, you can think of the diaphragm as either a belly bulger or a rib cage lifter (see figure 1.12). The muscular action of the diaphragm is most often associated with a bulging movement in the upper abdomen, which is commonly referred to as a belly breath or abdominal breath, and confusingly referred to as a diaphragmatic breath. This is only one type of diaphragmatic breath—one in which the base of the rib cage (lower attachments) is stable and the domes (upper attachments) are mobile (see figure 1.13a).

If we reverse these conditions by stabilizing the upper domes while relaxing the rib cage, a diaphragmatic contraction causes an expansion of the rib cage (see figure 1.13b). This is called a chest breath, which many believe to be caused by the action of muscles other than the diaphragm. This mistaken idea creates a false dichotomy between diaphragmatic and so-called "non-diaphragmatic" breathing.

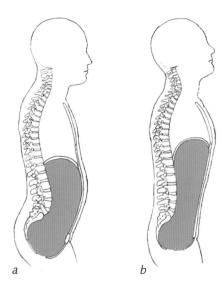

a   *b*

Figure 1.12   The diaphragm can be *(a)* a belly bulger during the belly inhalation, or *(b)* a rib cage lifter during the chest inhalation.

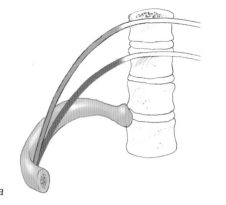 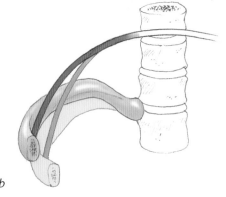

a   *b*

Figure 1.13   *(a)* With the rib cage stable and the abdominal muscles relaxed, the diaphragm's contraction lowers the upper attachments; *(b)* with the rib cage relaxed and the upper attachments stabilized by abdominal action, the contracting diaphragm lifts the rib cage upward.

The unfortunate result of this error is that many people receiving breath training who exhibit chest rather than belly movement are told that they are not using the diaphragm, which is entirely wrong. Except in cases of paralysis, the diaphragm is *always* used for breathing. The real issue is whether or not the diaphragm is able to work efficiently, meaning how well it can coordinate with all the other muscles that can affect shape change. Yoga practice can help with precisely this coordination.

If it were possible to release all of the muscular action surrounding our cavities, the diaphragm's action would cause both the chest and abdomen to move simultaneously. This rarely occurs because the need to stabilize the body's mass in gravity causes many of the respiratory stabilizing muscles—which are also postural muscles—to remain active through all phases of breathing, even while supine. From this perspective, our postural habits are synonymous with our breathing habits.

Engine of Three-Dimensional Shape Change

The specific patterns we encounter in yoga asana or breathing practice (pranayama) result from the action of accessory muscles—muscles other than the diaphragm—that can change the shape of the cavities. They have the same relationship to the diaphragm that the steering mechanism of a car has to its engine.

The engine is the prime mover of a car. All mechanical and electrical movements that are associated with a car's operation are generated by the engine. Similarly, three-dimensional, thoracoabdominal shape changes of breathing are primarily generated by the diaphragm.

When you drive, the only direct control you exert over the function of the engine is the speed of its spinning. Pushing the gas pedal makes the engine spin faster, and releasing the pedal makes it spin slower. When breathing, the only direct, volitional control you have over your diaphragm is its timing. Within limits you can control when it fires, but when it ceases contracting, a passive recoil creates the exhalation, just as your car's gas pedal springs upward to decelerate upon release of your foot.

Steering Shape Change

Everyone knows you don't steer a car with its engine. To channel the power of the engine in a particular direction, you need the transmission, brakes, steering, and suspension. In the same way, you don't steer your breathing with your diaphragm. To control the power of the breath and guide it into specific patterns, you need the assistance of accessory muscles.

From the standpoint of this engine analogy, the notion that improving breath function by training the diaphragm is flawed. After all, you don't become a better driver by learning how to work only the gas pedal. Most of the skills you acquire in driver training have to do with coordinating the acceleration of the car with steering, braking, and awareness of your surroundings. Likewise, breath training is really accessory muscle training. Only when all the musculature of the body is coordinated and integrated with the action of the diaphragm can breathing be efficient and effective.

The notion that diaphragmatic action is limited to abdominal bulging (belly breathing) is as inaccurate as asserting that an engine is only capable of moving the car forward and that some separate source of power governs reverse movement. This automotive error results from not understanding the relationship of the car's engine to its transmission; the breathing error results from not understanding the diaphragm's relationship to rib cage movement and to the accessory muscles.

A related error equates belly movement with proper breathing and chest movement with improper breathing. This is just as silly as stating that a car is best served by only going forward at all times. Driving a car with no reverse gear will eventually leave you stuck somewhere.

Accessory Muscles of Respiration

Although there is universal agreement that the diaphragm is the principle muscle of breathing, there are varied and sometimes conflicting ways of categorizing the other muscles that participate in breathing. By restating our definition of breathing, we can define as accessory muscles any muscle other than the diaphragm that can cause a shape change in the cavities. It is irrelevant whether shape change leads to inhalation (an increase of thoracic volume) or exhalation (a decrease in thoracic volume), because muscles that control both can be active during any phase of breathing.

Let's use this perspective to analyze the differences and similarities between a few types of breathing.

In a belly breath, the costal attachments of the diaphragm are stabilized by muscles that pull the rib cage downward: the internal intercostals, the transversus thoracis, and others (see figures 1.15 and 1.16 on the following page). These muscles are generally classified as exhaling muscles, but here they actively participate in shaping an inhalation.

In a chest breath, the upper attachments of the diaphragm are stabilized by the lower abdominal muscles, also regarded as exhaling muscles, but in this case, they clearly act to produce a pattern of inhaling. It should be noted that in both the chest and belly breaths, one region of accessory muscles had to be relaxed while the other was active. In the belly breath, the abdominal wall released, and in the chest breath, the so-called rib cage depressors had to let go.

In the cleansing technique of kapalabhati (kapala meaning skull and bhati meaning light or shine), in which strong, voluntary exhalations are the focus, the base of the rib cage needs to be lifted and held open in order to allow the lower abdominal region to freely, rhythmically change shape. Here the "inhaling" muscles of the external intercostals remain active during exhalation.

Abdominal and Thoracic Accessory Muscles

The abdominal cavity and its musculature can be imagined as a water balloon surrounded on all sides by elastic fibers running in all directions (figure 1.14).

In concert with diaphragmatic contractions, the shortening and lengthening of these fibers produce the infinitely variable shape changes associated with respiration. As the tone of the diaphragm increases during inhalation, the tone of some abdominal muscles must decrease to allow the diaphragm to move. If you contract all your abdominal muscles at once and try to inhale, you'll notice that it's quite difficult because you've limited the ability of your abdomen to change shape.

The abdominal muscle group does not affect breathing only by limiting or permitting shape change in the abdominal cavity. Because these muscles also attach directly to the rib cage, they directly affect its ability to change shape.

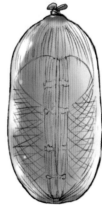

Figure 1.14 The shape-changing of the abdominal cavity (similar to a water balloon) is modulated by many layers of musculature running in all directions.

The abdominal muscles that have the most direct effect on breathing are the ones that attach at the same place as the diaphragm, the transversus abdominis. This deepest layer of the abdominal wall arises from the costal cartilage at the base of the rib cage's inner surface. The fibers of the transversus abdominis are interdigitated (interwoven) at right angles with those of the diaphragm, whose fibers ascend vertically, whereas those of the transversus abdominis run horizontally (see figure 1.15). This makes the transversus abdominis the direct antagonist to the diaphragm's action of expanding the rib cage. The same layer of horizontal fibers extends this action upward into the posterior thoracic wall as the tranversus thoracis, a depressor of the sternum.

The other layers of the abdominal wall have similar counterparts in the thoracic cavity. The external obliques turn into the external intercostals, and the internal obliques turn into the internal intercostals (see figure 1.16). Of all these thoracoabdominal layers of muscle, only the external intercostals are capable of increasing thoracic volume. All the others produce a reduction of thoracic volume, either by depressing the rib cage or pushing upward on the upper attachments of the diaphragm.

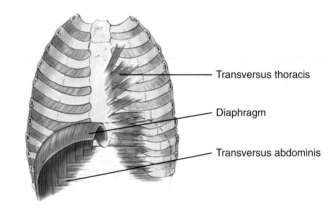

Figure 1.15 Posterior view of the chest wall, showing the interdigitated origins of the diaphragm and transversus abdominis forming perfect right angles with each other. This is clearly an agonist–antagonist, inhalation–exhalation muscle pairing that structurally underlies the yogic concepts of prana and apana.

Transversus thoracis

Diaphragm

Transversus abdominis

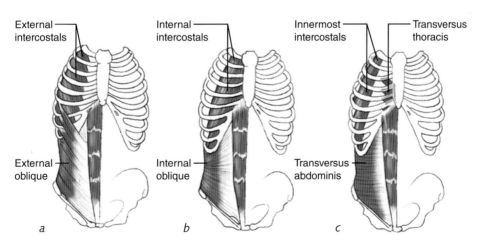

External intercostals

External oblique

Internal intercostals

Internal oblique

Innermost intercostals

Transversus abdominis

Transversus thoracis

a   *b*   *c*

Figure 1.16 The continuity of the abdominal and intercostal layers shows how *(a)* the external obliques turn into the external intercostals, *(b)* the internal obliques turn into the internal intercostals, and *(c)* the transversus abdominis turns into the transversus thoracis and innermost intercostals.

Other Accessory Muscles

Chest, neck, and back muscles can increase the volume of the rib cage (see figures 1.17 and 1.18), but they are far more inefficient at doing this than the diaphragm and external intercostals. This inefficiency is the result of the fact that the location and attachment of these muscles do not provide good leverage on the rib cage, and the usual role of these muscles is not respiration. They are primarily head, neck, shoulder girdle, and arm mobilizers—actions that require them to be stable proximally (toward the core of the body) and mobile distally (toward the periphery of the body). For these muscles to expand the rib cage, this relationship must be reversed; the distal insertions must be stabilized by yet more muscles so the proximal origins can be mobilized. That makes these the least efficient of the accessory muscles, and considering the degree of muscular tension that accessory breathing entails, the net payoff in oxygenation makes it a poor energetic investment. That is why improved breathing is observable as decreased tension in the accessory mechanism, which happens when the diaphragm, with its enormously efficient shape-changing ability, operates as unencumbered as possible.

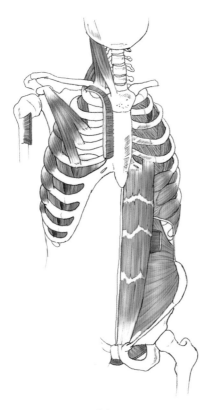

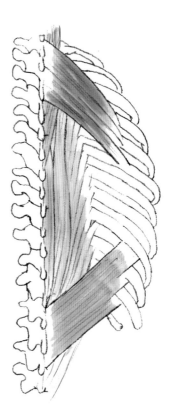

Figure 1.17   Some of the accessory muscles of respiration: Blue muscles act to reduce thoracic volume, while red muscles help to increase thoracic volume.

Figure 1.18   The serratus posterior muscles: Superior (red) assist thoracic volume increase; inferior (blue) assist thoracic volume reduction.

THE OTHER TWO DIAPHRAGMS

Along with the respiratory diaphragm, breathing involves the coordinated action of the pelvic and vocal diaphragms. Of particular interest to yoga practitioners is the action of *mula bandha*, or root lock (*mula* meaning firmly fixed or root, and *bandha* meaning binding, bonding, or tying), which is a lifting action produced in the pelvic floor muscles (shown in figure 1.19) that also includes the lower fibers of the deep abdominal layers. Mula bandha is an action that moves apana upward and stabilizes the upper attachments of the diaphragm. Inhaling while this bandha is active requires a release of the attachments of the upper abdominal wall, which permits the diaphragm to lift the base of the rib cage upward. This lifting action is referred to as *uddiyana bandha*, or flying upward lock.

It is important to note that the more superficial muscular fibers of the perineum need not be involved in mula bandha, because they are not efficient lifters of the pelvic floor. They also contain the anal and urethral sphincters, which are associated with the downward movement of apana (elimination of solid and liquid waste), as shown in figure 1.20.

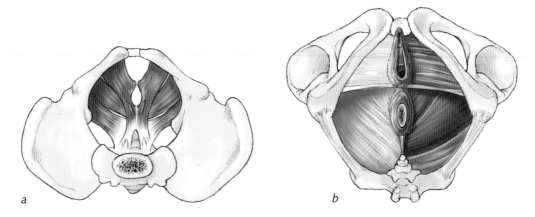

a　　　　　　　　　　　　　　　　　　　　　*b*

Figure 1.19 *(a)* The deepest muscles of the pelvic diaphragm, from above; *(b)* the pelvic floor from below, showing the orientation of superficial and deeper layers. The more superficial the layer, the more it runs from side to side (ischia to ischia); the deeper the layer, the more it runs front to back (pubic joint to coccyx).

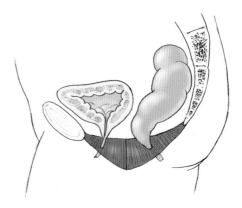

Figure 1.20 The action of the more superficial perineal fibers (see figure 1.19*b*) are associated with the anal and urogenital sphincters.

Vocal Diaphragm

The gateway to the respiratory passages is the glottis, shown in figure 1.21, which is not a structure but a space between the vocal folds (cords).

Yoga practitioners are accustomed to regulating this space in various ways based on what they are doing with their breath, voice, and posture. When at rest, the muscles that control the vocal cords can be relaxed so that the glottis is being neither restricted nor enlarged (see figure 1.22a). This occurs in sleep and in the more restful, restorative practices in yoga.

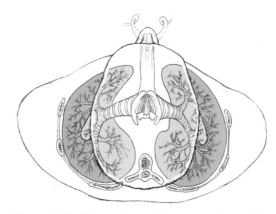

Figure 1.21   The pathway of air into and out of the lungs, showing the location of the vocal folds.

When doing breathing exercises that involve deep, rapid movements of breath, such as kapalabhati or bhastrika (*bhastra* meaning bellows) the muscles that pull the vocal folds apart (abduction) contract to create a larger passage for the air movements (see figure 1.22b).

When chanting, singing, or speaking, the vocal folds are drawn together (adduction), which causes them to vibrate as the exhaled air is forced across them. This vibration is termed *phonation* (see figure 1.22c).

When the exercises call for long, deep, slow breaths, the glottis can be partially closed, with only a small opening at the back of the cords (see figure 1.22d). This is the same

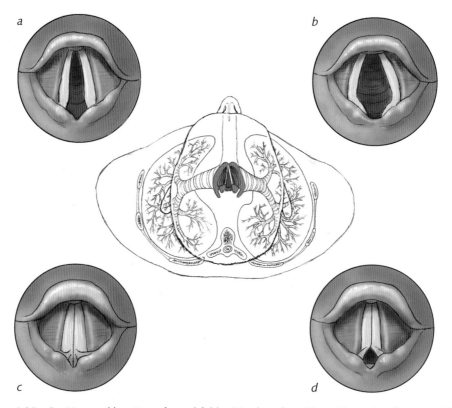

Figure 1.22   Position and location of vocal folds: *(a)* relaxed position, *(b)* maximally opened for forced respiration, *(c)* closed for speaking (phonation), *(d)* slightly opened for whispered speech (or *ujjayi*).

action that creates whispered speech; in yoga it's known as *ujjayi*, the victorious breath (*ud* meaning to flow out and *jaya* meaning victory or triumph). This action also creates more postural support in the body, as we will explore in the next section.

The Bandhas

All three diaphragms (pelvic, respiratory, and vocal) come together with ujjayi in yoga movements that are coordinated with inhaling and exhaling. In addition to giving more length and texture to the breath, the valve of ujjayi creates a kind of back pressure throughout the abdominal and thoracic cavities. This pressure can protect the spine during the long, slow flexion and extension movements that occur in the breath-synchronized flowing practice of *vinyasa* (arrangement or placement), such as during sun salutations. In yogic terms, these coordinated actions of the diaphragms (bandhas) create more sthira (stability) in the body, protecting it from injury by redistributing mechanical stress.

Figure 1.23 shows a mechanical analysis of the body entering into a forward bend from two perspectives. In figure 1.23*a*, we see the torso moving without breath support. Because the breathing musculature surrounding the cavities is not engaged, there is no single center of gravity to the shape, and a partial center of gravity (B) is acting upon the long arm of a lever (C), of which the fulcrum point (A) is at the vulnerable disc of the lumbosacral junction. The weight of the torso is being controlled by the posterior musculature, which compressively acts on the short end of the lever (D). The body instinctively resents this extremely poor leverage, and that's why we tend to hold our breath in situations like this to avoid damaging our spinal structures.

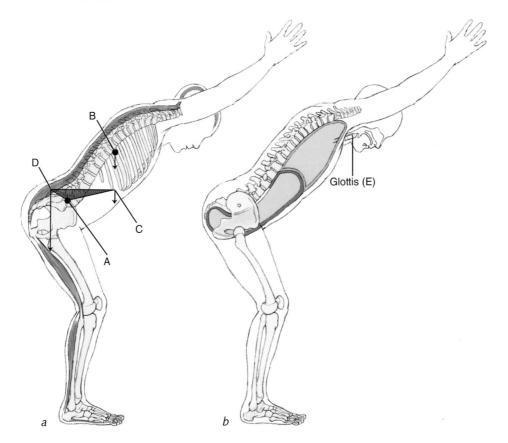

Figure 1.23   Supporting a movement *(a)* without the breath and *(b)* with the breath.

Figure 1.23b on page 19 pictures the same movement employing the glottal valve of ujjayi (E), which automatically engages the breathing musculature. This creates support along the entire anterior surface of the spine because it rests on the stabilized body cavities. The body now has a single center of gravity, which is being supported safely by the pelvis and legs. This is what is commonly referred to as frontal support.

An additional effect of moving and supporting the body through this kind of resistance is the creation of heat in the system, which can be used in many beneficial ways. These practices are referred to as brhmana (brh meaning increase or expand), which implies heat, expansion, and the development of power and strength as well as the ability to withstand stress. Brhmana is also associated with inhaling, nourishment, prana, and the chest region.

When relaxing the body in the more released, horizontal, or restorative practices, it is important to disengage the bandhas and glottal constrictions that are associated with vertical postural support. This relaxing side of yoga embodies the quality of langhana (meaning fasting or hunger), which is associated with coolness, condensation, relaxation, and release, as well as the development of sensitivity and inward focus. Langhana is also associated with exhaling, elimination, apana, and the abdominal region.

Because the ultimate goal of yoga breath training is to free up the system from habitual, dysfunctional restrictions, the first thing we need to do is free ourselves from the idea that there is a single correct way to breathe. As useful as the bandhas are when supporting the center of gravity and moving the spine through space, we need to release the brhmana forces of sthira in the system when pursuing the langhana, relaxation, and release of sukha.

INTRINSIC EQUILIBRIUM: PRESSURE ZONES

Intrinsic equilibrium refers to several important mechanisms that combine to make the human torso a self-supporting structure, which has an inherent tendency to seek upward movement.

The most important of these mechanisms is in the visceral component of the torso—the pressure differential between the lower abdomen (highest pressure), the upper abdomen (middle pressure), and the thoracic space (lowest pressure). Since energy always migrates from a region of higher pressure toward a region of lower pressure, this means that the lower and upper abdominal contents are constantly migrating upward toward thoracic space.[5]

The bony components of the torso—the spine, rib cage, and pelvis—all share a common characteristic: They are knit together under mechanical tension, like coiled springs restrained by elastic bands. When the sternum is divided for thoracic surgery, the two halves spring open and need to be pushed back together in order to be closed up again. At the front of the pelvis, the two pubic rami are joined at the pubic symphysis, a pressurized joint that softens and opens in childbirth and hopefully reknits afterward.

The spine's intervertebral discs are constantly pushing the vertebral bodies apart—an action that is resisted by the ligamentous and bony structures of the spine's posterior column. This combined push–pull of forces makes the spinal column as a whole a very springy structure that always seeks to return to neutral.

Note that all of these features of the body operate independently of muscle contraction—in fact, it is the unconscious, habitual activity of our postural and breathing musculature that obstructs the effect of intrinsic equilibrium. So, establishing an upright relationship to gravity, in the deepest sense, is less about exerting the correct muscular effort than it is about discovering and releasing the habitual muscular effort that is obstructing the natural tendency of the body to be supported all on its own.

---

[5] When a lobe of the lung is removed (lobectomy), the diaphragm and abdominal organs are drawn upward and fill the extra space.

This view of the body's anatomical support mechanisms is completely in harmony with the perspective on yoga practice offered by Patañjali. We achieve yoga by identifying and removing the kleshas (afflictions) from our system.

CONCLUSION

When translated, the term *pranayama* is commonly broken into the two roots *prana*, meaning life or breath energy, and *yama*, meaning restraint or control. Because the breath is only partially under our voluntary control, this translation gives a very limited view of breath practice.

A fuller understanding of the term is available when the second long "aa" (*pranaaayama*) is recognized. This means that the second root is *ayama*.

In Sanskrit, the prefix *a* negates the term it precedes. This means that pranayama refers to a process that *un*restrains the breath. It also honors the aspects of the breath that are not under our voluntary control.

This is why Patañjali's definition of kriya yoga (see page x in the introduction) so beautifully links with the idea that the breath is our best, most intimately available teacher of the deepest principles of yoga.

In this light, it is clear that the practice of unrestraining the breath can be seen as synonymous with the identification and release of the bodily tensions that obstruct the expression of our system's intrinsic equilibrium.

CHAPTER 2

YOGA AND THE SPINE

As the central nervous system, with its complex sensory and motor functions, evolved over millions of years and became absolutely essential to the survival of early humans, it required the corresponding development of one of nature's most elegant and intricate solutions to the dual demands of sthira and sukha: the spine. In order to understand how the human spine came to be what it is, we must first go back to studying the simple cell.

PHYLOGENY: A BRIEF HISTORY OF THE SPINE

Imagine the cell floating around in a primordial sea of fluid, surrounded by nutrients ready to be assimilated across its membrane (figure 1.1, page 2). Now imagine that the nutrients become less concentrated in some areas and more concentrated in others. The more successful organisms are the ones that develop the ability to reach the nutrients by changing their shape. This was probably the first form of locomotion; the pseudopod in figure 2.1 is an example of a simple cell with that ability. Shape changing as a survival method is an important principle to remember later on.

It is not too difficult to see how moving around becomes more and more valuable to these organisms, so the pseudopod eventually refines itself into a specialized organ, such as the flagella pictured in this bacterium (figure 2.2).

Now, rather than passively floating around in their environment, these primitive forms of life actively seek out nutrients that are necessary to their survival. An added benefit of mobility is that in addition to seeking out food, they can avoid becoming food for other organisms. Thus, we see the early biological basis for the yogic principles of raga and dvesha (attraction and repulsion). Seeking out the desirable and avoiding the undesirable is a fundamental activity of all living things, and another window into the concepts of prana and apana.

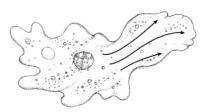

Figure 2.1 The cell changes shape and extends into a pseudopod.

Life forms respond to this pressure of seeking what's desirable and avoiding what's undesirable with ever more complex adaptations. As an organism's sensitivity and response to its surroundings become more complicated, it reaches a point where these activities require central organization and guidance.

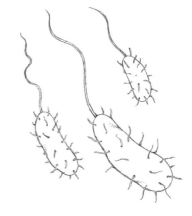

Figure 2.2 Bacterium with flagella.

Figure 2.3 shows a parasitic worm with a flattened body, called a *platyhelminth*, and in it we see the development of a rudimentary central nervous system. It exhibits a cluster of primitive nerve cells at the top and two nerve cords running down its length. Worms are invertebrates, but in their descendants, these rudimentary nerve cells have evolved into the brain, the spinal cord, and the dual trunks of the autonomic nervous system. They all require the corresponding development of a structure that allows for free movement but is stable enough to offer protection to these vital yet delicate tissues—in other words, a skeletal spine.

A central nervous system allows for an enormous amount of flexibility in a vertebrate's survival activities, and the spine must thoroughly protect it while still allowing free movement. In sea creatures such as the fish (figure 2.4), the shape of the spine is consistent with its environment: water surrounding on all sides, exerting an equal amount of mechanical pressure from top to bottom and side to side. As the fish employs its head, tail, and fins to propel itself through the water, the spinal movements are oriented in the side-to-side dimension.

Figure 2.3 A platyhelminth worm, with its rudimentary central nervous system.

This lateral undulation in the spine was preserved even when aquatic creatures made the enormous evolutionary leap to terrestrial life. Figure 2.5 demonstrates that pattern in the amphibious salamander. Even though its limbs (evolved from fins) are assisting in locomotion, they are not supporting the weight of the spine off the ground. That development, probably resulting from a need to orient the eyes to ever more distant food or threats, requires a dramatic reorientation of the spinal structures.

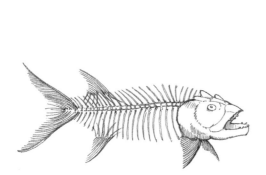

Figure 2.4 Fish with a straight spine.

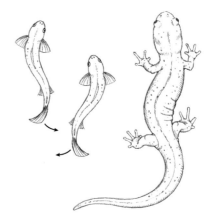

Figure 2.5 Lateral movements in both aquatic and amphibious spines.

A straight spine, such as that of the fish if it were supported on four limbs, would be subjected to gravity's maximum destabilizing force at its very weakest point: the center of the span between the two supported ends (figure 2.6). Once raised up on its limbs, the most successful newly terrestrial creatures would be those that arched their spines in response to gravitational stress in order to direct that stress toward the supported ends, rather than the unsupported middle.[1] This is the development of the primary curve of the terrestrial spine—what we know as our thoracic curve. It is primary in the sense that it is the first anterioposterior (front–back) curve to emerge, and also in the sense that it is the first curve that a human spine exhibits prenatally.

The curve of the neck was the next to evolve. Our fish ancestors had no real necks; their heads and bodies moved as a single unit with the gills placed directly behind the brain. The gradual downward shift of the breathing structures allowed for the development of a highly mobile neck that was capable of producing quick, precise movements of the head and sensory organs, offering an ever further look into its environment and tremendous survival advantages. This orientation of the cervical region signaled the first development of a secondary, or lordotic curve in the spine, which can be seen in the cat (figure 2.7).

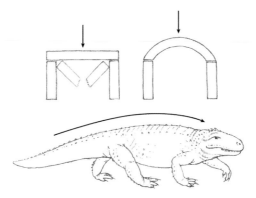

Figure 2.6   A supported arch is more stable than a straight line.

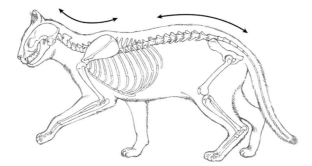

Figure 2.7   The first secondary curve: the cervical.

---

[1] Think of the difference between Greek and Roman architecture. Far more of the Romans' buildings are still standing because they built with arches and the Greeks didn't.

When creatures began to use their forelimbs to interact with their environment, the ability to bear weight on the lower extremities became more necessary, and this signaled the beginning of the uniquely human second lordotic curve—the lumbar. At first, it was just a flattening out of the primary curve at the base of the spine, in order to allow animals such as the yellow-bellied marmots pictured in figure 2.8 to support their center of gravity above their base of support for longer periods of time.

The presence of a tail also helped in that feat of balance, but as the tail gradually disappeared, the shape of the spine had to change in order to bring the center of gravity fully above the base of support. When this occurred in human evolution, the hip, sacral, and leg structures essentially remained stationary in their quadruped relationship to the earth, and the torso pushed its way up and back, forming the lumbar curve.

Figure 2.9a illustrates the difference in shape between a chimpanzee spine and a human spine. Notice the absence of a lumbar curve in the chimp. This is why in order to move across the ground, primates walk on their knuckles (figure 2.9b), and when they run on their hind legs, they must throw their long arms back. Without a lumbar curve, that is the only way they can get their weight over their feet.

The human spine is unique among all mammals in that it exhibits a full complement of both primary (thoracic and sacral) and secondary (cervical and lumbar) curves (figure 2.10).

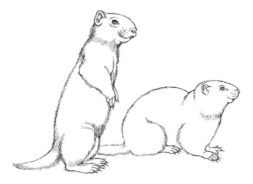

Figure 2.8   Flattening the primary curve to get the forelimbs off the ground.

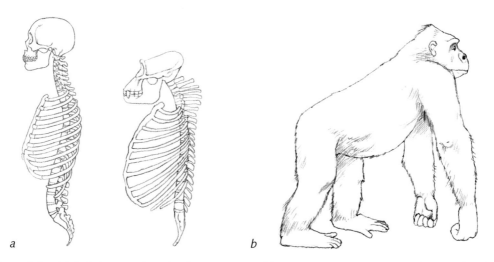

a   b

Figure 2.9   *(a)* Only humans have lumbar curves, so *(b)* our primate cousins cannot be considered true bipeds.

Only a true biped requires both pairs of curves; our tree-swinging and knuckle-walking cousins have some cervical curve but no lumbar curve, which is why they are not true bipeds.

If we view our evolution from quadruped to biped in yogic terms, we could say that the lower body developed more sthira for weight bearing and locomotion, and the upper body more sukha for breathing, reaching, and grasping. One way to describe it is that the lower body moves us out into the environment, while the upper body brings our environment in to us.

ONTOGENY: AN EVEN BRIEFER HISTORY OF OUR OWN SPINE

After understanding the evolution of our species (phylogeny), it is useful to study the developmental stages experienced by each individual human (ontogeny).

Although the developing fetus exhibits—and then loses—certain characteristics that we share with our ancient ancestors, such as gills and a tail, the theory that ontogeny recapitulates phylogeny has long since been discredited. There is, however, at least one sense in which this is true: how the phyolgenetic and ontogenetic development of our spines mirror each other. Consider how our fetal spines exhibit only the primary curve along their entire length; this remains the case for our entire intrauterine existence (figure 2.11).

The first time our spine moves out of that primary curve is when our heads negotiate the hairpin curve of the birth canal, and the neck experiences its secondary (lordotic) curve for the very first time (figure 2.12).

As our postural development proceeds from the head downward, the cervical curve continues to emerge after we learn to hold up the weight of our head at about 3 to 4 months and then fully forms at around 9 months, when we learn to sit upright.

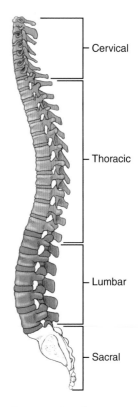

Figure 2.10 The curves of the spinal column.

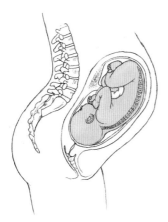

Figure 2.11 The entire spine exhibiting the primary curve in utero.

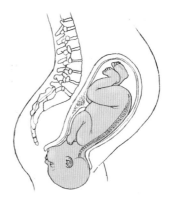

Figure 2.12 The first emergence of the secondary curve: negotiating the 90-degree turn from the cervix into the vaginal passage.

After crawling and creeping like our quadruped ancestors, in order to bring our weight over our feet we must acquire a lumbar curve. So, at 12 to 18 months, as we begin to walk, the lumbar spine straightens out from its primary, kyphotic curve. By 3 years of age, the lumbar spine begins to become concave forward (lordotic), although this is not outwardly visible until 6 to 8 years of age. After the age of 10, the lumbar curve fully assumes its adult shape (figure 2.13).

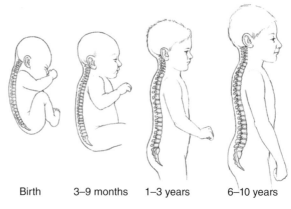

Birth   3–9 months   1–3 years   6–10 years

Figure 2.13 Development of primary and secondary curves.

The full glory of nature's ingenuity is apparent in the human spine, perhaps even more so than in other vertebrates. From an engineering perspective it is clear that we have the smallest base of support, the highest center of gravity, and the heaviest cranium (proportional to our total body weight) of any other mammal. As the only true bipeds on the planet, we are also earth's least mechanically stable creatures. Fortunately, the disadvantage of having a cranium as heavy as a bowling ball balancing on top of the whole system is offset by the advantage of having that big brain; it can figure out how to make it all work efficiently, and that's where yoga can help.

Our human form in general, and our spines in particular, exhibit an extraordinary resolution between the contradictory requirements of rigidity and plasticity. As we shall see in the next section, the structural balancing of the forces of sthira and sukha in our living bodies relates to the principle of intrinsic equilibrium, the deep source of support that can be uncovered through yoga practice.

ELEMENTS OF LINKAGE BETWEEN THE VERTEBRAE

The spinal column as a whole is ideally constructed to neutralize the combination of compressive and tensile forces to which it is constantly subjected by gravity and movement. The 24 vertebrae are bound to each other with intervening zones of cartilaginous discs, capsular joints, and spinal ligaments (shown schematically in blue in figure 2.14). This alternation of bony and soft tissue structure represents a distinction between passive and active elements; the vertebrae are the passive, stable elements (sthira), and the active, moving elements (sukha) are the intervertebral discs, facet (capsular) joints, and a network of ligaments that connect the arches of adjacent vertebrae (figure 2.15). The intrinsic equilibrium of the spinal column can be found in the integration and interaction of these passive and active elements.

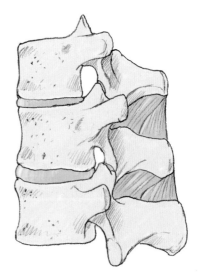

Figure 2.14 Alternating zones of hard and soft tissue in the spinal column.

To understand the overall architecture of the spine, it is useful to view it as two separate columns. In the schematic side view in figure 2.16, its front-to-back dimension can be roughly divided in half between a column of vertebral bodies and a column of arches. Functionally, this arrangement very clearly evolved to contend with the dual requirements of stability and plasticity. The anterior column of vertebral bodies deals with weight-bearing, compressive forces, whereas the posterior column of arches deals with the tensile forces generated by movement. Within each column, the dynamic relationship of bone to soft tissue exhibits a balance of sthira and sukha. The vertebral bodies transmit compressive forces to the discs, which resist compression by pushing back. The column of arches transmits tension forces to all the attached ligaments (figure 2.17), which resist stretching by pulling back. In short, the structural elements of the spinal column are involved in an intricate dance that protects the central nervous system by neutralizing the forces of tension and compression.

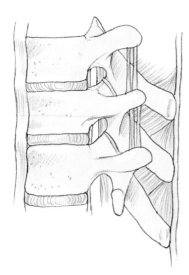

Figure 2.15   Ligaments of the spine.

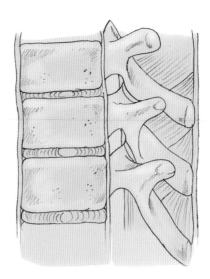

Figure 2.16   Side view of the spine divided into an anterior column of vertebral bodies and discs, and a posterior column of arches and processes.

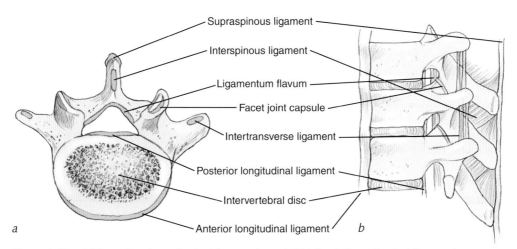

Supraspinous ligament

Interspinous ligament

Ligamentum flavum

Facet joint capsule

Intertransverse ligament

Posterior longitudinal ligament

Intervertebral disc

Anterior longitudinal ligament

a

b

Figure 2.17   *(a)* Superior view of spinal ligaments and *(b)* lateral view of spinal ligaments.

Discs and Ligaments

If you look deeper, you can also see how sthira and sukha are revealed in the components of an intervertebral disc: The tough, fibrous layers of the annulus fibrosis tightly enclose the soft, spherical nucleus pulposus. In a healthy disc, the nucleus is completely contained all around by the annulus fibrosis and the vertebra (see figure 2.18). The annulus fibrosis is itself contained front and back by the anterior and posterior longitudinal ligaments, with which it is closely bonded (see figure 2.17 on page 29).

This tightly contained arrangement results in a strong tendency for the nucleus to always return to the center of the disc, no matter in which direction the body's movements propel it.

From the top of the cervical spine to the base of the lumbar spine, individual vertebrae are dramatically different in shape based on the functional demands of the varying regions of the spine (figure 2.19). There are, however, common elements to all vertebral structures, as illustrated by the schematic representation in figure 2.20.

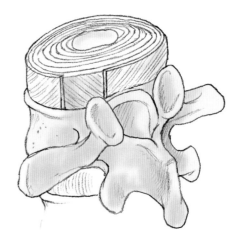

Figure 2.18 The nucleus pulposus is tightly bound by the annulus fibrosis, which contains concentric rings of oblique fibers that alternate their direction in a manner similar to that of the internal and external obliques of the abdominals.

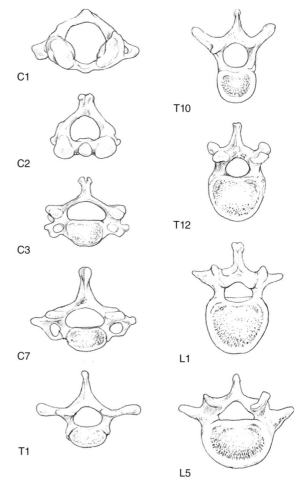

Figure 2.19 Form follows function: the changing shape of the vertebrae.

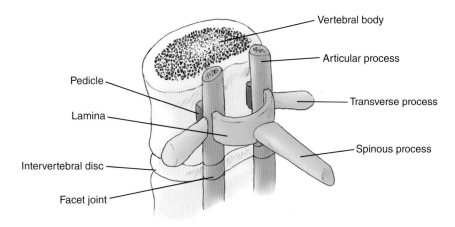

Figure 2.20   Common elements of a vertebra's structure.

Weight-bearing activities in general, as well as axial rotation (twisting movements), produce symmetrical (axial) compressive forces that flatten the nucleus into the annulus, which pushes back, resulting in a decompressive reaction (see figure 2.21). If the compressive force is high enough, rather than rupture, the nucleus loses some of its moisture to the porous bone of the vertebral body. When the weight is taken off the spine, the hydrophilic nucleus draws the water back in, and the disc returns to its original thickness. That is why humans are a bit taller right after getting out of bed.

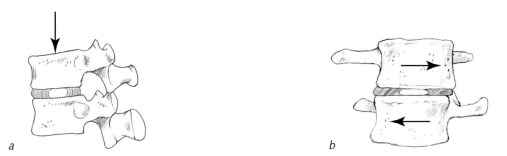

a   b

Figure 2.21   (a) Weight-bearing forces as well as (b) twisting produce symmetrical compression (flattening) of the nucleus, which, under pressure from the annulus, returns to its spherical shape, thus decompressing the vertebrae.

Push–Counterpush

The movements of flexion, extension, and lateral flexion produce asymmetrical movements of the nucleus, but the result is the same: Wherever the vertebral bodies move toward each other, the nucleus is pushed in the opposite direction, where it meets the counterpush of the annulus, which causes the nucleus to push the vertebral bodies back to neutral (see figure 2.22).

Assisting in this counterpush are the long ligaments that run the entire length of the spine, front and back. The anterior longitudinal ligament runs all the way from the upper front of the sacrum to the front of the occiput, and it is fixed tightly to the front surface of each intervertebral disc. When it is stretched during backward bending, not only does it tend to spring the body back to neutral, but the increased tension at its attachment to the disc also helps to propel the nucleus back to neutral. The opposite action occurs in the posterior longitudinal ligament when it is stretched in a forward bend. It runs from the back of the sacrum to the back of the occiput.

Every movement that produces disc compression in the anterior column necessarily results in tension to corresponding ligaments attached to the posterior column. The recoiling of these ligaments out of their stretched state adds to the other forces of intrinsic equilibrium, which combine to return the spine to neutral.

Note that all this activity occurs in tissues that behave independently of the circulatory, muscular, and voluntary nervous systems. In other words, their actions do not impose an energy demand on these other systems.

a   b

Figure 2.22   *(a)* Flexion and *(b)* extension movements produce asymmetrical movements of the nucleus, which, under pressure from the annulus, returns to a central position, thus helping the spine to return to neutral.

TYPES OF SPINAL MOVEMENT

There are generally thought to be four possible movements of the spine: flexion, extension, axial rotation (twisting), and lateral flexion (side bending). These four movements occur more or less spontaneously in the course of daily life: bending over to tie your shoes (flexion; see figure 2.23), reaching for something on a high shelf (extension; see figure 2.23), grabbing a bag in the car seat behind you (axial rotation; see figure 2.24 on page 34), or reaching your arm into the sleeve of an overcoat (lateral flexion; see figures 2.25 and 2.26 on pages 35 and 36). There are, of course, yoga postures that emphasize these movements as well. What follows is a detailed analysis of these ranges of motion. Please note that these ranges are averages established by measuring a wide variety of people. Any given individual will exhibit significant variations at both ends of the spectrum of flexibility and in differing regions of their spines. The numbers given for degrees of range of motion are approximate, as are the angles pictured, with a five degree variation in either direction.

	Extension	Flexion	Total
Cervical	75°	40°	115°
Thoracic	25°	45°	70°
Lumbar	35°	60°	95°
Total	135°	145°	280°

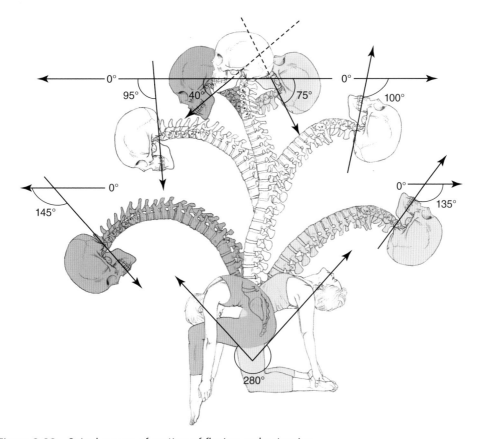

Figure 2.23 Spinal ranges of motion of flexion and extension.

Adapted from *Physiology of the Joints, Vol. 3: The Vertebral Column, Pelvic Girdle and Head, 6th Edition,* A.I. Kapandji, page 39, copyright 2008, with permission from Elsevier.

	Axial rotation
Cervical	50°
Thoracic	35°
Lumbar	5°
Total	90°

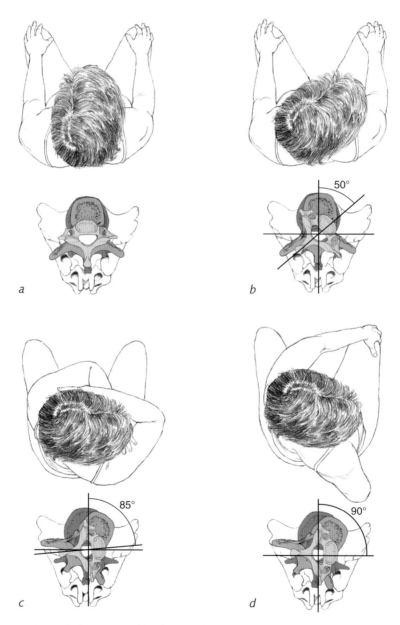

Figure 2.24   Cervical, thoracic, and lumbar axial rotation: *(a)* neutral, 0 degrees axial rotation; *(b)* cervical only, 50 degrees axial rotation; *(c)* cervical plus thoracic, 85 degrees axial rotation; and *(d)* cervical plus thoracic plus lumbar, 90 degrees axial rotation.

	Lateral flexion
Cervical	35°
Thoracic	20°
Lumbar	20°
Total	75°

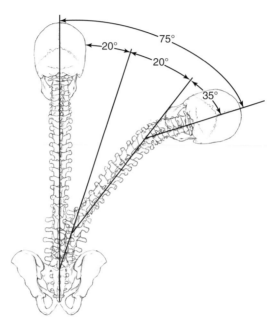

Figure 2.25 Spinal ranges of motion of lateral flexion. Note how the 75 degrees of lateral flexion is the movement most evenly distributed throughout the spine.

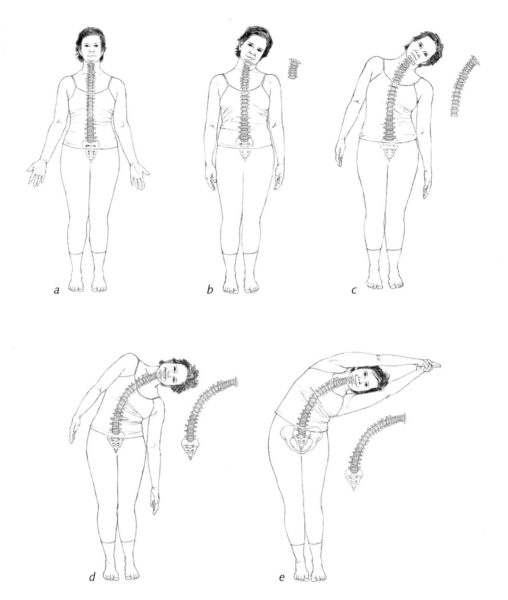

Figure 2.26 *(a)* Neutral spine; *(b)* cervical lateral flexion; *(c)* cervical and thoracic lateral flexion; *(d)* cervical, thoracic, and lumbar lateral flexion; and *(e)* lateral flexion and lateral pelvic shift.

A more thorough look into the nature of the four ranges of motion of the spine shows that a fifth possibility called axial extension exists. This motion does not happen spontaneously in the normal course of daily movements. You have to learn how to make it happen intentionally because it is somewhat "unnatural" (see page 42).

Flexion and Extension, the Primary and Secondary Curves, and Inhalation and Exhalation

The most basic movement of the spine emphasizes its primary curve: flexion. As discussed previously, the primary curve is the curve present primarily in the thoracic spine, but it is also obvious in the shape of the sacrum. It is no accident that the yoga pose that most commonly exemplifies spinal flexion is called child's pose (see figure 2.27)—it replicates the primary curve of the unborn child. From a certain perspective, all the curves of the body that are posteriorly convex can be seen as reflections of the primary curve. A simple way to identify all the primary curves is to notice all the parts of the body that contact the floor in savasana, or corpse pose (see figures 2.28 and 2.29): the curve of the back of the head, the upper back, the sacrum, and the backs of the thighs, the calves, and the heels. Consequently, the secondary curves are present in all the body parts that are off the floor in this position: the cervical and lumbar spine, the backs of the knees, and the space posterior to the Achilles tendons.

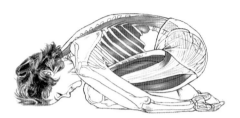

Figure 2.27   Child's pose replicates the primary curve of the unborn child.

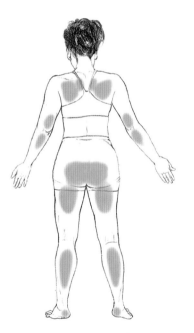

Figure 2.28   In corpse pose, the primary curves of the body (blue shaded areas) contact the floor.

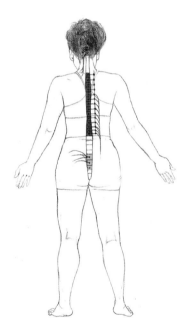

Figure 2.29   Corpse pose seen from below, showing spinal origins of the autonomic nervous system—sympathetic from the thoracic region and parasympathetic from the cervical and sacral regions.

From this perspective, spinal flexion can be defined as an increase in the primary spinal curves and a decrease in the secondary spinal curves. A reversal of this definition would define spinal extension as an increase in the secondary curves and a decrease in the primary curves.

Note that as far as movement is concerned, the relationship between the primary and secondary curves is reciprocal: The more you increase or decrease one, the more the other wants to do the opposite. For example, an increase in the thoracic curve automatically produces a decrease in the cervical and lumbar curves.

A classic yoga exercise that explores this reciprocal relationship of the primary and secondary curves is cat–cow, or chakravakasana (see figure 2.30).

Supported at both ends by the arms and thighs, the spine's curves can move freely in both directions, producing the shape changes of flexion and extension. Although it is common for instructors to teach this movement by telling the student to exhale on spinal flexion and inhale on spinal extension, it is more accurate to say that the shape change of spinal flexion *is* an exhalation and the shape change of spinal extension *is* an inhalation. As our definition of breathing shows, spinal shape change is synonymous with breathing shape change.

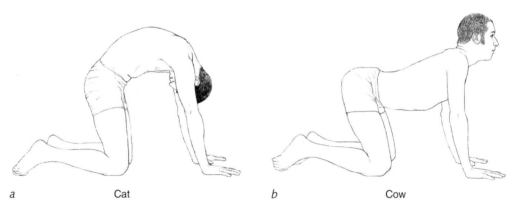

a   Cat   b   Cow

Figure 2.30 The cat–cow exercise emphasizes both the *(a)* primary and *(b)* secondary curves.

MOVEMENT EXPLORATION

From a comfortable sitting position, try increasing your thoracic curve by dropping your chest forward. Notice how your neck and lower back flatten. Now, try the same movement, but initiate it with your head; if you drop your head forward, you'll notice how the chest and lower spine will follow. The same will occur if you initiate this movement with your lower spine. You may also notice that these flexion movements of the spine generally tend to create an exhalation.

Going in the opposite direction, try decreasing your thoracic curve by lifting your chest. Notice how your neck and lower back increase their curves. If you try initiating the movement with your head or lower spine, the results will be the same. Did you notice if these extension movements of the spine tend to create an inhalation?

Spatial Versus Spinal Perspectives in Forward- and Backward-Bending Poses

Spinal extension is not necessarily the same thing as bending backward, and spinal flexion is not necessarily the same thing as bending forward. To avoid confusion, it is important to keep these distinctions clear. Flexion and extension refer to the relationship of the spinal curves to each other, while forward bending and backward bending are terms that refer to movements of the body in space. The terms are not necessarily interchangeable. By way of illustration, consider the following contrasting examples of how two different body types might appear in some standard yoga movements.

1. A stiff, sedentary office worker, whose stooped posture doesn't change as his hips move forward and his arms reach overhead in an attempt to do a standing back bend: His spine remains in flexion while his body moves backward in space (figure 2.31a).

2. A flexible dancer, who hyperextends her spinal curves in the overhead reach and keeps her spine extended as she flexes forward at the hip joints to move into uttanasana (standing forward bend): Her spine remains in extension while her body bends forward in space (figure 2.31b).

The valuable skill in observing movements this way is the ability to distinguish movement of the spinal curves in relation to each other from the movements of the torso in space.

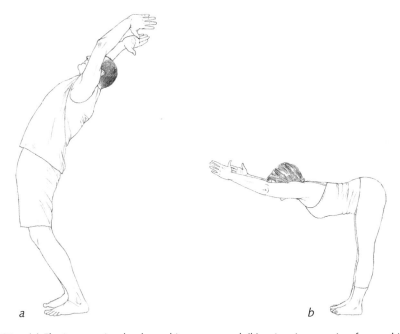

a   b

Figure 2.31 *(a)* Flexion moving backward in space, and *(b)* extension moving forward in space.

Figure 2.32 shows more of an integrated orientation to a standing back bend. Here, the secondary curves are kept under control, and the pelvis is kept firmly over the feet. As a result, there is much less movement backward in space, but a greater emphasis on thoracic extension (reduction of the primary curve). Although this is not a dramatic movement spatially, it actually provides a safe and effective stretch to the thoracic and rib structures and is less disturbing to the process of breathing than either the dancer's or the office worker's movements.

Spatial Versus Spinal Perspectives in Lateral and Twisting Movements

When looking at yoga poses that involve lateral and twisting movements, it is also important to distinguish spatial from spinal perspectives. Trikonasana, or triangle pose, is often referred to as a lateral stretch, and this is true insofar as it lengthens the connective tissue pathway that runs along the side of the body (see figure 2.33).

However, it is possible to lengthen the lateral line of the body without any appreciable lateral flexion of the spine, so again, it must be clear what exactly is meant by the term *lateral bend*.

In trikonasana, more of a lateral line stretch would result from a wide spacing of the feet, and an intention to initiate the movement primarily from the pelvis while maintaining the spine in neutral extension. This also turns the pose into more of a hip opener.

Lateral flexion of the spine could be emphasized by a closer spacing of the feet. This allows for more stabilization of the relationship between the pelvis and thighs, which would require the movement to come from the lateral bending of the spine.

When we look at parivrtta trikonasana, the revolved variation of triangle pose (figure 2.34*a*), we can apply the same perspective to the twisting action of the spine. The lumbar spine is almost entirely incapable of axial rotation (only 5 degrees; see figure 2.34*b*), which, in this

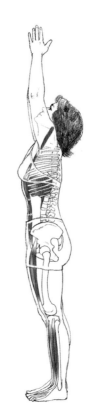

Figure 2.32   An integrated orientation to standing spinal extension without backward spatial movement.

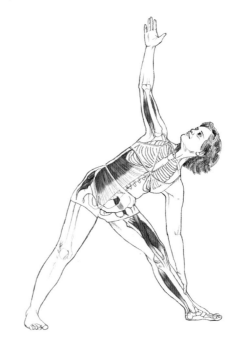

Figure 2.33   Lateral spatial movement with minimal lateral spinal flexion.

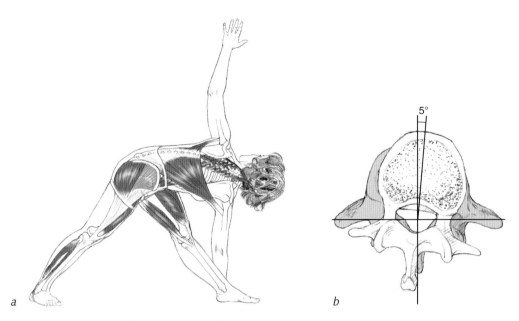

Figure 2.34 *(a)* Parivrtta trikonasana; *(b)* the entire lumbar spine can only twist 5 degrees around its vertical axis.

pose, means that it will go wherever the sacrum leads it. Consequently, for the lower spine to twist in the direction of this pose, the pelvis would have to turn in the same direction.

If the pelvis is free to rotate around the hip joints, this pose exhibits a more evenly distributed twist throughout the spine rather than an overloading of T11 and T12—the first joints above the sacrum that can freely rotate (see figure 2.35). The lumbar spine fully participates because the pelvis and sacrum are also turning; the neck and shoulders are free and the rib cage, upper back, and neck are open, along with the breathing.

If the hips are restricted, the lumbar spine appears to be moving in the opposite direction of the rib cage and shoulder girdle rotation. When this is the case, most of the twisting originates from T11 to T12 and above. In addition, the twisting of the shoulder girdle around the rib cage can create the illusion that the spine is twisting more than it really is. So, the body can indeed be twisting in space, but a careful observation of the spine may tell where exactly the twisting is coming from.

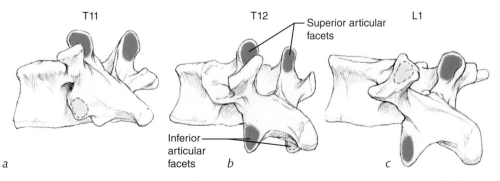

Figure 2.35 *(a-c)* T12 is a transitional vertebra. The inferior articular facets of T12 are lumbar, and where they articulate with the superior facets of L1, they do not permit axial rotation, while the superior articular facets of T12 are thoracic, which do. Therefore, the T11 and T12 articulations are the first spinal joints above the sacrum that can freely rotate. (Facets in light blue are hidden from view.)

Axial Extension, Bandhas, and Mahamudra

The fifth spinal movement, axial extension, is defined as a simultaneous reduction of both the primary and secondary curves of the spine (see figure 2.36). In other words, the cervical, thoracic, and lumbar curves are all reduced, and the result is that the overall length of the spine is increased.

Because the primary and secondary curves have a reciprocal relationship, which is expressed in the natural movements of flexion and extension, axial extension is "unnatural" in the sense that it bypasses this reciprocal relationship by reducing all three curves at once. In other words, axial extension generally doesn't happen all on its own; it usually requires conscious effort and training to accomplish.

The action that produces axial extension involves a shift in the tone and orientation of the breathing structures known as the bandhas. The three diaphragms (pelvic, respiratory, and vocal) and their surrounding musculature become more sthira (stable). As a result, the shape-changing ability of the thoracic and abdominal cavities is more limited in axial extension. The overall effect is a reduction of breath volume but an increase in length. The overall yogic term that describes this state of the spine and breath is *mahamudra*, or great seal, which always involves axial extension and the bandhas. It is possible to do mahamudra from many positions, including seated, standing, supine, and in arm support.

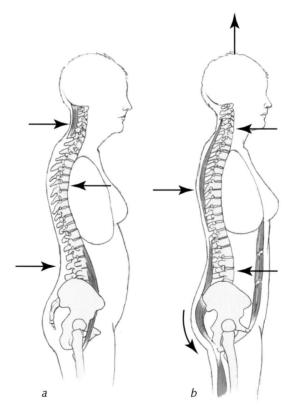

a   *b*

Figure 2.36 Axial extension involves a simultaneous reduction of *(a)* the primary and secondary curves, which *(b)* lengthens the spinal column beyond its neutral alignment.

A seated posture named *mahamudra* (figure 2.37) adds a twisting action to axial extension. It is considered a supreme accomplishment to do this practice with all three bandhas executed correctly, because it represents a complete merging of asana and pranayama practice.

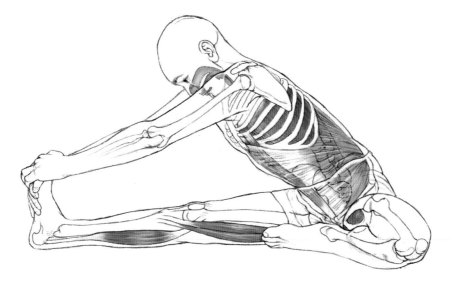

Figure 2.37 Mahamudra combines axial extension, a twisting action, and all three bandhas.

INTRINSIC EQUILIBRIUM:
THE SPINE, RIB CAGE, AND PELVIS

If you were to remove all the muscles that attach to the spine, it still would not collapse. Why? Intrinsic equilibrium is the concept that explains not only why the spine is a self-supporting structure but also why any spinal movement produces potential energy that returns the spine to neutral. The same arrangement exists in the rib cage and pelvis, which, like the spine, are bound together under mechanical tension. Intrinsic equilibrium is also exhibited by the pressure zone differentials described in the previous chapter (page 20).

These facts about the core structures of the axial body reveal a deeper truth about how yoga practice appears to liberate potential energy from the body.

True to the principles of yoga and yoga therapy, the most profound changes occur when the forces obstructing that change are reduced. In the case of intrinsic equilibrium, a deep level of built-in support for the core of the body is involved. This built-in support does not depend on muscular effort because it is derived from the relationships among the noncontractile tissues of cartilage, ligament, and bone. Consequently, when this support asserts itself, it is always because some extraneous muscular effort has ceased to obstruct it.

It takes a lot of energy to fuel our constant, unconscious muscular exertions against gravity, and that is why the release of that effort is associated with a feeling of liberated energy. Thus, it is tempting to refer to intrinsic equilibrium as a source of energy because its discovery is always accompanied by a profound sensation of increased vitality in the body. In short, yoga can help to release the stored potential energy of the axial skeleton by identifying and releasing the less efficient extraneous muscular effort that can obstruct the expression of those deeper forces.

CONCLUSION

As noted at the end of chapter 1, a balance of both will and surrender is needed in order to honor the true nature of the breath and the spine in yoga practice. Without this perspective, the deeper, intrinsic support within the system is forever overshadowed by a futile attempt to reproduce through effort what nature has already placed at the core of the body.

Every system of the body is involved in every movement we make. Without the active participation of the nervous, circulatory, endocrine, respiratory, digestive, immune, connective tissue, fluid, skeletal, ligamentous, and muscular systems (to mention just a few), we wouldn't be able to create the movements of the breath or lift our arms overhead and fold forward into uttanasana, much less launch the body through space into a handstand.

DYNAMIC BALANCE OF BODY SYSTEMS

Any part of the body that we turn our attention to is part of more than one system: While bones are generally considered part of the skeletal system, they also play important roles in other systems, such as the circulatory, nervous, immune, and endocrine systems. The bones are part of the circulatory and immune systems because red and white blood cells are created in the bone marrow. They are part of the nervous system because of the role calcium has in the working of neurons, and they are part of the endocrine system because of the hormones secreted by bone cells that play a role in our metabolism. None of these systems can work alone. Without the circulatory system, other systems such as the respiratory, endocrine, and digestive systems would not be able to distribute oxygen, hormones, and nutrients to the cells of the body. Without the nervous system, it would be impossible to coordinate the muscles of the limbs or to modulate the dilation of the blood vessels to supply the bones, brain, heart, or muscles with enough blood. All of the systems of the body are overlapping and interdependent (figure 3.1, page 46).

If we focus on just one or two systems in studying anatomy and yoga, we run the risk of terribly oversimplifying the incredible effects that the practice of asana has on every system in the body. On the other hand, we can dive deeply into a single point of focus and find incredible complexity that enriches our experience of the whole. For the purposes of this book, the focus is on the role of the skeletal and muscular systems in generating the movements that create asana, knowing that starting at any beginning point can bring us into a relationship with all the other systems and tissues in the body.

MUSCULOSKELETAL SYSTEM

Bones, ligaments, muscles, and tendons all weave together into a dynamic whole. The skeletal portion of the musculoskeletal system is made up of the bones, ligaments, and other tissues that make up the joints: synovial fluid, hyaline cartilage, and fibrocartilaginous discs and wedges. The muscular portion is made up of the muscles and tendons that cross the joint space and attach to the bones, as well as the nerve endings that organize the exquisite sequencing and timing of our muscle actions. All of these tissues are either composed of or wrapped in layers of connective tissue.

The skeletal system and the muscular system are often treated as separate systems. When we consider how movement is generated, it makes more sense to think of them as one musculoskeletal (or skeletomuscular) system. The muscles and bones work intimately together to negotiate our relationships to gravity and space, to provide our upright posture, and to help us move through the world, feed ourselves, use tools, and create change.

Without the structure and support of the skeletal system, the muscles would be a puddle of contractile tissue with nothing to move. On the other hand, without the movement

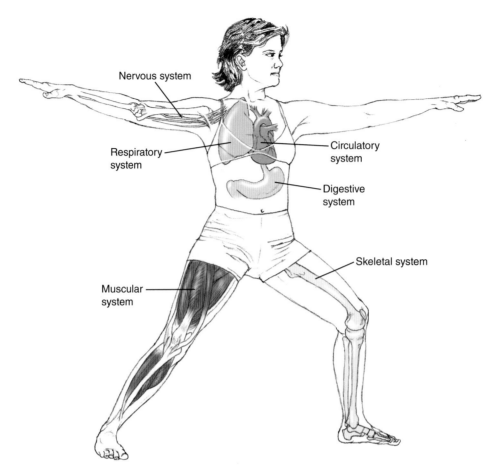

Figure 3.1 Several systems of the body: nervous, digestive, respiratory, circulatory, skeletal, and muscular.

created by muscles, the bones would be unable to move through space and could only respond to forces outside the body travelling through them. Without connective tissue such as ligaments and tendons, bones and muscles would have no way to relate to each other.

One job of the bones is to receive weight and transmit force, while the ligaments direct that force along specific pathways. This weight and force might be generated by the pull of gravity or by other sources, such as the muscles that propel the leg through space to take a step. The job of the muscular system is to move the bones into positions where they can do their job as effectively as possible.

SKELETAL SYSTEM TISSUE: BONES AND LIGAMENTS

Our bones are incredible structures. They are strong enough to resist collapsing under the force we send through them, light enough that we can move them through space, and resilient enough to adapt to stresses that come from all directions in three-dimensional space.

Ligaments do an amazing job as well. They are flexible enough to allow three-dimensional movement at the joint and strong enough to align and guide a tremendous amount of force from bone to bone across the space of the joint.

Movement in the skeletal system happens on many levels. On a cellular level, individual cells are constantly breaking down and building up the matrix of the bone and the fibers of ligaments. On a tissue level, each bone and ligament has some degree of ability to change shape in response to the forces travelling through it. On a system level, movement happens where a relationship exists between two or more bones: the joints.

JOINTS

In the skeletal system the term *joint* describes the space where the surfaces of two or more bones come into relationship and *articulate* with each other. A joint is more of an event than a place in the sense that it depends on movement and change for its existence. If any movement is happening, however miniscule, then there is a joint.

Conventionally, joints are classified structurally by the tissue that connects the two bones. This could be cartilage, fibrous tissue, synovial fluid, or some combination of the three. Joints can also be classified functionally by the degree of movement possible and biomechanically by the number of bones involved and the complexity of the joint.

In the analysis of asana, we observe movement in synovial joints, the most mobile joints in the body. (Several of these synovial joints are also at least partly cartilaginous or fibrous.)

Synovial Joints

Starting from the center and moving outward, a synovial joint is composed of the bones that articulate with each other, the synovial fluid between them, the membrane that creates that synovial fluid, and the connective tissue that surrounds and protects the whole structure (figure 3.2).

To be more specific, the articulating surfaces at the ends of the bones are covered with a layer of hyaline cartilage that cushions and protects. These layers of hyaline cartilage are slippery and allow the ends of the bones to slide along each other with little friction.

Between these layers of hyaline cartilage, synovial fluid acts as a lubricant and facilitates the sliding of the articulating surfaces. Synovial fluid also distributes force in the joint to a slight degree, and it acts as a fluid seal between the two surfaces, as oil does between two panes of glass, holding them together. Synovial fluid is secreted by a synovial membrane (or *synovium*) that is connected to both bones. The presence of this synovial membrane defines the boundaries of the joint space: Everything outside the synovial membrane is outside the joint space.

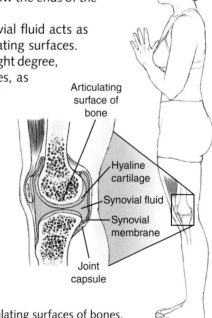

Articulating surface of bone

Hyaline cartilage

Synovial fluid

Synovial membrane

Joint capsule

Figure 3.2 All synovial joints have the following: articulating surfaces of bones, hyaline cartilage, synovial fluid, a synovial membrane (synovium), and a joint capsule (not pictured but present in an actual knee joint is the meniscus).

The synovial membrane is wrapped by layers of connective tissue that form the joint capsule, providing containment for the movement possibilities created by the mobility of the hyaline cartilage and synovial fluid. On the very outside of the joint capsule are fibers that thicken and organize themselves into straplike bands, the collateral ligaments. These ligaments direct the force that travels through a joint and keep the movement on track.

Superficial to all these elements are the muscles that travel across the joint.

Balanced Joint Space

In a healthy, functional joint, the space between the two bones is balanced, and maintains that balance throughout the full range of motion (ROM) in that joint. Balance is not the same as symmetry, and maintaining balanced joint space[1] through the range of motion doesn't mean that the joint space is evenly distributed at absolutely every moment.

Balanced joint space is instead the product of a complex set of factors, including but not limited to the contours of the articulating surfaces of the bones, the viscosity of the synovial fluid, the resilience of the joint capsule and ligaments around the joint, and the assorted contractions of the muscles around the joint. In a larger sense, the hydration of the tissues, the efficiency of the circulatory system, the ability of the nervous system to sense movement in the joint, and the quality of the mind's attention contribute to this balance.

The layer of hyaline cartilage at the end of each bone is able to absorb a tremendous amount of force and distribute that force into the trabeculae, the weight-bearing scaffolding of the bone. This force then travels through bone and joint and bone and joint until it meets a surface that can absorb the force, such as the earth, or it is discharged in some movement through space, such as throwing a ball. That force could also be received and transmitted to another structure, or dispersed in unhelpful ways through soft tissues.

When the joint space is not balanced through the full range of movement and force is not distributed across the articulating surfaces, there is some wear and tear on the hyaline cartilage. Like other tissues in the body, the hyaline cartilage constantly remodels itself and can repair minor wear and tear without long-term consequences. (There are other tissues in the body, such as muscles, that remodel at a faster rate than the hyaline cartilage.) If the imbalance in the joint space is consistent and continuous over a long period of time, the hyaline cartilage cannot repair itself and can eventually become damaged or worn away. If the hyaline cartilage is worn away, the ends of the bones rub against each other. This friction eventually stimulates the bones to grow unevenly, which causes more friction and stress on the bones. This cycle of friction and growth can become quite painful and is one cause of osteoarthritis.

Lack of balance in the joint space can arise for a variety of reasons. Sometimes people are just born with joints that don't line up efficiently. More often the challenge arises from inefficient movement patterns that eventually lead to imbalances in the joint capsule and ligaments, over- or underuse of the muscles surrounding the joint, or habitual patterns in the nervous system. These habits are often perpetuated through familiarity and lack of awareness. Even a perfectly appropriate idea, exercise, or image can be dangerous when done for too long or in a way that excludes any other ideas. Our ideas about movement are at fault as much as the bones and ligaments we are born with. For example, pulling the shoulders back to open up the front of the chest is a common instruction. This is a

---

[1] I first learned the concept of balanced joint space through Body–Mind Centering (BMC). It is fundamental to BMC's approach to repatterning movement in the skeletal and ligamentous systems.

useful instruction for people whose shoulders have slid forward around their rib cage. If, however, there is an issue in the spine, pulling the shoulders back might increase neck and upper back effort without addressing the underlying spinal issue. Also, it might be an effective instruction once or twice, but if someone continues to pull the shoulders back for an extended period of time, that person will end up pulled so far back that he is out of balance in the other direction.

Joint Actions

It is a fundamental fallacy to think that our human bodies work like the structures that humans have built. Human joints are frequently compared to devices used in construction to create joints, such as a hinge or a ball and socket. The mechanics of a human joint, however, are not the same as those of a joint between pieces of wood or metal or ceramic or plastic, in part because of the nature of the materials.[2]

Useful as it might be on a superficial level to compare the workings of the elbow joint to a hinge, drawing this parallel limits our ideas about how movement happens at the joint. Nothing in the body is perfectly flat or straight or less than three-dimensional, including the articulating surfaces of the bones. Because these articular surfaces always have volume and contour, movement in the joints is always three-dimensional.

The conventional terms used to describe movement at the joints, *joint actions*, describe fairly simple movements that are flat and two-dimensional and happen in a single plane. No single joint action takes into account the volume of the movement possibilities at every joint.

The implication of using two-dimensional language to describe movement at our joints is that we simplify our concept of what movements are possible and then simplify the movements we do. The danger is that we deprive ourselves of movement choices and overuse the few options we think are available to us.

Because all the articulating surfaces in our joints are three-dimensional, every joint is capable of more than one joint action, if not three or four. Equal amounts of movement are not possible in each action, but even if it is a tiny movement, the joint has movement in every dimension. That tiny movement could have huge repercussions on two or three joints or in 5 to 10 years down the line.

Conventional Definitions of Joint Actions

The basic terms that describe joint actions apply to a majority of the joints in the body. Several terms have specific meanings in particular joints, and some terms are used in more than one joint but mean different things in different joints.

Anatomical definitions of joint actions often use planes to describe the movement. A plane is a two-dimensional surface, and the three basic planes intersect at right angles to each other. When the planes are oriented so that they intersect in the center of the body, they can be used to describe relationships within the body (anterior and posterior describe a sagittal relationship of body parts) or movements (flexion and extension describe sagittal movement of the spine). The *vertical plane* (also called the coronal or door plane) divides the body into front and back. The *horizontal plane* (also called the transverse or table plane) divides the body into top and bottom. The *sagittal plane* (also called the median or wheel plane) divides the body into right and left sides.

---

[2] If you are interested in reading more about these differences, Steven Vogel has written a fascinating book called *Cats' Paws and Catapults: Mechanical Worlds of Nature and People* (W. W. Norton & Company, 1998).

Spinal Joint Actions

The following terms describe movements when the joints of the spine are moving and the vertebrae articulate in relationship to each other. In these spinal actions the actual shape of the spine changes, which is a different action than moving the spine through space (by articulating at the hips, for example, which would be an action in the legs). Common yoga language such as *forward bending* is a nonanatomical description that can refer to either a movement of the spine through space or the spinal joint action of flexion (see chapter 2, page 33).

flexion—Movement in the sagittal plane that brings the anterior surfaces of the body toward each other.

extension—Movement in the sagittal plane that brings the anterior surfaces of the body away from each other.

lateral flexion—Movement in the vertical or coronal plane that bends the spine to one side or the other.

rotation—Movement in the horizontal or transverse plane, around the vertical axis of the spine:

- In **rolling,** all of the parts of the spine rotate in the same direction.

- In **twisting,** one part of the spine turns a different direction from another part of the spine.

axial extension—Movement along the vertical axis of the spine that lengthens the spine by taking out the sagittal curves.

circumduction—Movement that travels through space around the axis of the body, tracing a cone shape. This is not the same as rotation.

Limb Joint Actions

These terms describe the joint actions that can happen in the upper and lower limbs, which include the shoulder girdle and pelvis. As in the spine, there is a difference between moving a joint through space and actually articulating in the joint, which is the joint action. (For example, when you lift your whole arm to the ceiling, the elbow does move through space but it doesn't necessarily articulate.)

Actions in All Limbs

For the joint actions below, the same terms can be used to describe movement at a variety of joints. Which bones are involved in the movement will depend on which joint is articulating.

flexion—Movement in which the anterior surfaces of the limb move toward each other; depending on the position of the spine, hips, and shoulders, this could happen in any plane. Because of a spiral in the limbs that occurs while we are embryos, flexion in the knee, ankle, and foot joints moves what we consider the back surfaces of the leg toward each other.

extension—Movement in which the anterior surfaces move away from each other; again, depending on the position of the spine, hips, and shoulders, this could happen in any plane. And, because of that embryological spiral, extension in the knee, ankle, and foot joints moves what we consider the back surfaces of the leg away from each other.

rotation—Movement around the axis of the limb; in the hips, shoulders, and forelegs, this is further described as internal (or medial) and external (or lateral) rotation. Rotation in the hand, foot, and forearm has special names (see the sections that follow).

abduction—Movement of the limb away from the torso or the midline of the body; in the hand, foot, and scapula, this term describes a more specific action (see the sections that follow).

adduction—Movement of the limb toward the torso or the midline of the body; in the hand, foot, and scapula this term describes a more specific action (see sections that follow).

circumduction—Movement that travels through space around the axis of the limb, tracing a cone shape. This is not the same as rotation.

Actions in Specific Limbs

Some parts of the limbs can perform movements that are not described by the general terms listed above. These joint actions have terms that are used for specific body parts (such as *pronation* and *supination*, which only occur in the feet and forearms, or *radial deviation*, which only occurs in the wrists). In some body parts a general joint action will refer to a different movement than in the rest of the limb. (In the hands, abduction refers to movement away from the middle finger rather than away from the midline of the body.)

Hand

rotation—Rotation around the long axis of the hand is called **eversion** when it lifts the outer edge of the hand and **inversion** when it lifts the inner edge of the hand.

abduction—Movement of the fingers away from the third finger.

adduction—Movement of the fingers toward the third finger.

radial deviation—Movement of the fingers toward the radial (thumb) side of the hand.

ulnar deviation—Movement of the fingers toward the ulnar (pinkie) side of the hand.

opposition—Movement of the thumb and the little finger toward each other.

Wrist

dorsiflexion—Movement when the angle between the back of the hand (the dorsal surface) and the forearm decreases. (From an embryological perspective, this is extension of the wrist.)

palmar flexion—Movement when the angle between the palm of the hand (the palmar surface) and the forearm decreases. (From an embryological perspective, this is flexion of the wrist.)

radial deviation or abduction—Movement of the hand toward the radial side of the forearm (thumb side).

ulnar deviation or adduction—Movement of the hand toward the ulnar side of the forearm (pinkie side).

Forearm

rotation—Rotation of the radius and ulna so that they cross each other is called **pronation,** and rotation of the radius and ulna so that they are uncrossed is called **supination.** (Sometimes pronation is described as "palm down" and supination as "palm up," but the position of the palm doesn't accurately describe these actions because of the movements available in the shoulder joint and scapula.)

Clavicle

elevation—Movement of the distal end of the clavicle upward in the vertical plane.

depression—Movement of the distal end of the clavicle downward in the vertical plane.

upward rotation—Rotation of the clavicle around its longitudinal axis to roll the top surface backward.

downward rotation—Rotation of the clavicle around its longitudinal axis to roll the top surface forward.

protraction—Movement of the distal end of the clavicle forward, usually accompanied by scapular protraction.

retraction—Movement of the distal end of the clavicle backward, usually accompanied by scapular retraction.

Shoulder (Glenohumeral Joint)

flexion—Movement of the arm sagittally forward in space.

extension—Movement of the arm sagittally backward in space.

abduction—Movement of the arm from alongside the torso to open to the side and away from the body.

adduction—Movement of the arm from an abducted position toward the side of the body.

horizontal abduction—Movement of the arm from a flexed position in front of the body to open to the side and away from the body.

horizontal adduction—Movement of the arm from an abducted position to the side of the body to a flexed position in front of the body.

protraction—Movement that slides the head of the humerus forward in the sagittal plane.

retraction—Movement that slides the head of the humerus backward in the sagittal plane.

Scapula

elevation—Sliding of the scapula upward in the vertical plane.

depression—Sliding of the scapula downward in the vertical plane.

upward or lateral rotation—Rotation of the scapula in the vertical plane in such a way that the glenoid fossa faces upward and the inferior angle moves laterally to the side.

downward or medial rotation—Rotation of the scapula in the vertical plane in such a way that the glenoid fossa faces downward and the inferior angle moves medially toward the spine.

abduction or protraction—Movement in the horizontal plane away from the spine, which ends up wrapping the scapula toward the front of the body.

adduction or retraction—Movement in the horizontal plane toward the spine, which ends up drawing the scapulae toward each other in the back.

Foot

rotation—Rotation around the long axis of the foot is called **eversion** when it lifts the outer edge of the foot and **inversion** when it lifts the inner edge of the foot.

abduction—Movement of the forefoot toward the lateral edge (little toe side) of the foot without moving the heel; the movement of the toes away from the second toe.

adduction—Movement of the forefoot toward the medial edge (big toe side) of the foot without moving the heel; the movement of the toes toward the second toe.

pronation and supination—In the feet, **pronation** is sometimes considered the same thing as **eversion**, and is sometimes a combination of **eversion** and **abduction**. And in the feet, **supination** is sometimes used interchangeably with **inversion**, and is sometimes a combination of **inversion** and **adduction**.

Ankle

plantar flexion—Movement when the angle between the sole of the foot (the plantar surface) and the back of the foreleg decreases; pointing the foot. (From an embryological perspective, this is ankle flexion.)

dorsiflexion—Movement when the angle between the top of the foot (the dorsal surface) and the foreleg decreases. (From an embryological perspective, this is ankle extension.)

Pelvis

nutation—Movement of the sacrum separately from the pelvic bones in such a way that the top of the sacrum tips forward, or nods, and the bottom of the sacrum (near the coccyx) tips back. This is movement at the sacroiliac (SI) joint, between the sacrum and pelvic or innominate bone, not movement of the full pelvis (which would be an anterior or posterior tilt of the pelvis caused by joint action at the hip joints or lumbar spine).

counternutation—Movement of the sacrum in such a way that the top of the sacrum tips backward and the bottom of the sacrum (near the coccyx) tips forward. This is movement at the SI joint, between the sacrum and innominate bone, not movement of the full pelvis (which would be an anterior or posterior tilt of the pelvis caused by joint action at the hip joints or lumbar spine).

Range of Motion in Joints

The body never moves only one joint or does only one joint action. In any given movement, the body might be moving through the subtleties of 15 or even 500 different joint actions just to bend a leg or lift an arm.

Even if we set out to completely focus on one particular joint, as soon as we begin a movement, it travels to the joints at the other ends of the moving bones and into the next bones and joints and the next bones and joints and the next—all the way into the spine and all the way out to the periphery. If you are lying passively and someone else moves you, that movement will still travel through your tissues one way or another.

Because movement travels through the body in this way, it isn't practical to focus exclusively on the range of motion in a single joint. While it is possible for a skilled hands-on practitioner to effectively isolate a joint and determine how much movement is possible in the bones and soft tissues, as soon as we begin to move volitionally, we must take into account the rest of the movement choices in the body.

In observing the wholeness of a person moving, you are able see that when movement seems to stop in one joint, it moves to the next. Sometimes it skips over joints that don't move easily or becomes so small that it is difficult to perceive, but it always goes somewhere.

Instead of focusing on the range of motion in specific joints, look at the whole pattern of movement in the skeletal system: Observe where there is much movement and it seems easy, and observe where there is less movement and it seems more challenging. Then ask how to bring balance: If someone has made it to the limit of what can happen in one joint, is movement possible at the next joint? Do some joints do all the movement to the point of being overly mobile? Are some joints not moving at all, as if there aren't joints there? It can also be a question of attention: Whether someone is very flexible or very stiff, his or her body will have places where there is a lot of awareness and places that are more in the shadows.

CONCLUSION

Success in an asana (or any movement) should be measured by the quality of balance or intrinsic equilibrium through the whole body, rather than in the range of motion in a single joint. This quality arises in the skeletal system from the presence of balanced joint space in each joint, the availability of clear pathways for movement through the bones and joints, and the awareness of our individual patterns in the wholeness of the systems of our body.

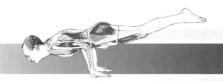

If the job of the skeletal system is to transfer weight and force by way of the ligaments through the bones in any arrangement the joints allow, then the task of the muscular system is to move the bones into place so that the bones can do their job. Muscles create movement, joints enable movement, and connective tissue translates movement from tissue to tissue. Bones absorb and transmit movement, and nerves coordinate and organize the whole gorgeous dance.

The muscles work together as a matrix of potential movement choices. This matrix affects every articulation in the body. Muscles do not work in isolation, and a single muscle never works without support and modulation from other muscles. Each muscle has an effect on every other muscle, whether they are nearby or far away.

Historically, muscles have been presented in a simplistic, linear paradigm, which leads to misconceptions such as:

- Muscles work as discrete units.
- For every body, the same muscles always create the same joint action.
- The more tone a muscle has, the better it can function.
- Muscles always relate to each other in the same way.
- There is a correct set of muscles for executing any movement.

To understand why these assumptions are incorrect, it is necessary to examine the basic anatomy of muscles.

BASIC MUSCLE ANATOMY

What we usually think of as a working muscle is actually an organ made up of at least four different tissues: muscle tissue, connective tissue, nerves, and blood vessels (figure 4.1, page 56). The muscle tissue itself has the ability to contract and create movement. The connective tissue communicates the power of that contraction to whatever the muscle is connected to, such as bones, organs, or skin. The nerves tell the muscle when to fire, for how long, and at what intensity, and the blood vessels provide the nourishment that allows the muscle tissue to be active.

Muscles are divided into three basic types: skeletal muscle, cardiac muscle, and smooth muscle.

Try this experiment: Lie down on your back. Open your arms to the sides at a comfortable level, palms facing up. Your legs can be bent or extended. Take some time to settle into this position. Then, starting with a very small movement, begin to wiggle your fingers.

Can you feel how the muscles in your forearms are activated as you wiggle your fingers? How about the muscles in your upper arms? The muscles in your shoulders and upper back? Can you feel the muscles around your spine respond to the wiggling of your fingers? How about the muscles in your jaw? Can you follow the movement to your feet?

If it feels as though the movement doesn't travel anywhere, see if you can feel where it stops. Are you holding on to anything in your muscles that you don't need to? What can you release so that the movement can travel with ease through the body?

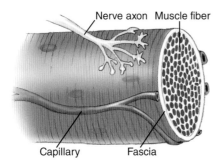

Figure 4.1 Muscles are composed of several tissues working together: muscle fibers, nerves, capillaries (blood vessels), and fascia (connective tissue).

Skeletal muscle is generally attached to bones and creates movement at the joints. It has alternating bands of light and dark fibers that give the tissue its striated appearance. Skeletal muscle is controlled by the somatic portion of the nervous system, which makes many of its functions voluntary, or under our conscious control. Cardiac muscle is in the heart, and smooth muscle is in the blood vessels, airways, and visceral organs. Cardiac tissue is also striated but is controlled by the autonomic nervous system and hormones from the endocrine system. Smooth muscle is not striated and, like cardiac muscle, is controlled by the autonomic nervous system and the endocrine system.

The skeletal muscle tissue that we see with the naked eye is made up of bundles of fascicles. The fascicles are made up of bundles of muscle fibers, which are the actual muscle cells. Inside the muscle cells are bundles of myofibrils (or myofilaments; see figure 4.2). Each of these bundles of myofibrils, muscle cells, and fascicles are wrapped in a layer of connective tissue, and all these layers of connective tissue come together at the ends of the muscles to create the tendons and other tissues that connect muscles to bones (figure 4.3).

The myofibrils are made up of thick and thin filaments that lie alongside each other and overlap. These filaments are twisted strands of molecules that create contractions.

Figure 4.2 The muscle belly is made up of bundles of fascicles that are made up of bundles of fibers (muscle cells) containing bundles of myofibrils.

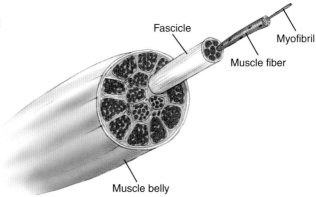

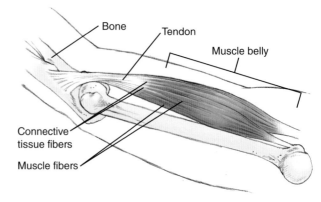

Figure 4.3 Fibers of connective tissue (white) run through the muscle (red). At either end of the muscle, the connective tissue comes together to create tendons, which connect to bone.

MUSCLE CONTRACTIONS

When a muscle cell contracts, the molecules create and release bonds between the thick and thin filaments, which ratchet along each other and create a sliding movement that increases their overlap and draws the two ends of the myofibril toward each other. If enough myofibrils shorten, the whole muscle fiber slides shorter. As more and more muscle fibers contract, they attempt to shorten the entire muscle by sliding the attachment points at the two ends of the muscle toward each other.

Whether or not the entire muscle does actually shorten depends on outside factors, specifically how much resistance exists. If only a few filaments are sliding together inside the cells, they may not generate enough force to overcome the weight of whatever structure the muscle is attached to, such as the weight of the arm or the weight of the head. The weight of a body part is a product of the resistance created by gravity, which is a fundamental source of resistance for everything on this planet. We negotiate this force every time we lift an arm, stand up, roll over, or take a breath. Added resistance also comes from other forces, such as the weight of something being carried, an opposing muscle contraction, or even an emotional state (for example, tension, anger, or the effort not to cry will often create resistance, while relaxation, happiness, or relief will often decrease resistance).

Muscles do not contract in an all-or-nothing way. All of the fibers do not have to contract at the same time, meaning that a muscle can generate a precisely graded amount of force, coordinated by the dialogue between the nervous system and the muscles. Because muscles work in this modulated way, they don't always end up shortening, even though the fibers might be actively contracting. A muscle may in fact be active and lengthening when the outside force is greater than the force that the muscle is exerting.

The words *concentric*, *eccentric*, and *isometric* are used to describe muscle actions (figure 4.4, page 58). These terms actually describe the effects of the relationship between the muscle and the resistance it meets.

Concentric Contraction   The muscle fibers contract and generate *more* force than the resistance that is present so that the ends of the muscle slide toward each other and the muscle shortens.

Eccentric Contraction   The muscle fibers contract and generate *less* force than the resistance that is present so that the ends of the muscle slide apart and the muscle actually lengthens. The muscle is active as it lengthens, so this is not the same as relaxing the muscle.

Isometric Contraction   The muscle fibers contract and generate the *same* amount of force as the resistance that is present so that the ends of the muscle neither move apart nor move together and the length of the muscle does not change. Isometric contractions can be distinguished further: There is a difference in experience between intending to hold still against the resistance of something else trying to move you and intending to move but not being able to overcome the resistance to movement. There is also a difference in experience between maintaining an isometric contraction following a concentric contraction and maintaining an isometric contraction following an eccentric contraction.

> Muscles don't actually flex or extend; these terms describe joint actions. To be accurate, muscles use contractions to create all joint actions, including flexion and extension.

A relaxed muscle generally means that there is not an intentional or voluntary contraction of the muscle fibers. If someone is conscious (even sleeping), however, there is always an underlying level of automatic activity in the muscle fibers to maintain the resting tone of the muscle. This resting tone keeps the muscles ready to respond and in postural muscles automatically adjusts for slight shifts in weight and balance when we sit, stand, and walk.

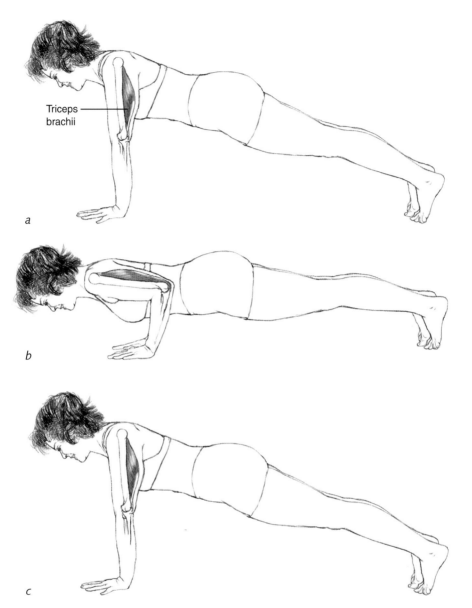

Triceps brachii

a

b

c

Figure 4.4 Examples of isometric, eccentric, and concentric contractions in the triceps brachii when (*a* to *b*) moving from plank to chatturanga (eccentric), (*b* to *c*) returning to plank from chatturanga (concentric), and (*a* and *c*) maintaining plank (isometric).

In the fields of fitness and movement training, the words *lengthen* and *stretch* are used in many different ways. It is important to understand that a muscle can lengthen and be active (an eccentric contraction), can lengthen and be inactive (a relaxed muscle), or can lengthen and gradually change from active to inactive or vice versa.

In any of these situations, the muscle lengthens because an outside force (such as the pull of gravity or the pull of another muscle) acts more strongly than the muscle being lengthened. Lengthening a muscle does not necessarily mean relaxing it.

The word *stretch* is sometimes used interchangeably with *lengthen*. If the term simply means to change the distance between the attachment points of the muscle in such a way that they move apart from each other, *stretch* is indeed interchangeable with *lengthen*.

If, however, *stretch* implies a particular quality of sensation in the muscle, then it is not interchangeable with *lengthen*. It is possible to lengthen a muscle without a stretching sensation—in fact, most of us do it all the time. Actions such as walking, talking, or picking up a cup all involve lengthening and shortening muscles, often without any particular muscular sensation at all.

ORIGIN AND INSERTION FALLACY

The places where muscles attach to the bones are often classified as being the *origin* and the *insertion*. The origin is the attachment that is closer to the torso or the center of the body, and the insertion is the attachment that is farther from the center, closer to the fingers, toes, skull, or coccyx. The underlying implication is that the origin is the fixed point and the insertion is the point that moves; however, this is only true for some of our movements. Any time we move the torso through space, we reverse the so-called origin and insertion points.

This classification of attachment points also implies that muscles develop from one point to another and they somehow grow from the origin toward the insertion. Embryologically, however, they do not do this. Instead, clusters of future muscle cells migrate to the area of their future home and organize themselves once they get there. It is not a linear point-to-point process at all.

MUSCLE RELATIONSHIPS

No muscle works in isolation; all muscles in the intricate web of the muscular system constantly engage with each other to balance, reinforce, modify, and modulate one another through the matrix of the connective tissue.

The relationships between muscles can be organized in a variety of ways. We can focus on how muscles balance each other around a single joint, how the layers of muscle have different effects as they shift from deep to superficial, or how kinetic chains of muscle and connective tissue integrate the limbs and torso.

Agonist–Antagonist Pairs

One of the common paradigms for organizing muscles is into agonist–antagonist muscle pairs. This perspective is oriented around specific joint actions and the muscles that create and modulate those joint actions.

The starting place is a specific joint, the focal joint, and a specific joint action. For every joint action there are muscles that create the movement and muscles that oppose the movement. The muscles that create the joint action are called the agonists, or prime movers, and the muscles that create the opposite joint action are called the antagonists.[1] These pairs of agonist–antagonist muscles can have direct relationships in the nervous system at the level of the spinal cord. When one muscle of the pair acts, the other muscle receives a message to respond and modulate. This relationship is called reciprocal innervation or reciprocal inhibition. Not all agonist–antagonist muscle pairs have a relationship at the level of the spinal cord; some are paired together through repeated movement patterns that are recorded at higher levels in the brain rather than the spinal cord.

---

[1] The word *agonist* comes from a Greek word meaning contender or contestant. *Antagonist* comes from the Greek word for opponent.

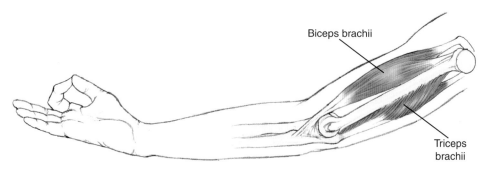

Figure 4.5 When the focal joint is the elbow and the joint action is flexion against gravity, the biceps brachii is the agonist and the triceps brachii is the antagonist.

Agonist and antagonist roles are relative, and they change as the focal joint and the joint action change. These terms do not describe an absolute quality inherent in the muscle itself but something about its relationship to another muscle during a specific moment at a particular joint. Whether a muscle is an antagonist or an agonist depends on which joint and which joint action are the points of focus and where the main resistance to the movement is found (figure 4.5).

The muscles that support and modulate the action of the agonist or antagonist muscles are called synergistic muscles. The synergistic muscles also act to minimize excess movement at a joint or to stabilize one part of the body to support movement in another part. When synergists act to stabilize in this way, they are also called fixators. Alternatively, the term *synergistic* is used to describe a whole group of muscles that work together to create an action. Synergistic muscles are essential for maintaining balanced joint space and for the health of the joint.

Organizing muscles into agonist–antagonist pairs is very useful when looking at a specific action at a single focal joint. In order to consider how different joints relate to each other, it is important to examine other kinds of relationships between muscles.

Sometimes, even in a simple movement, the antagonist for the first part of the movement becomes the agonist in the second part of the movement. For example, when the arm is extended out to the side, parallel to the floor, and the elbow is flexed so that the hand moves toward the shoulder, in the first part of the movement (bringing the forearm perpendicular to the floor), the triceps brachii is an antagonist to the action of the biceps brachii. In the second part of the movement (bringing the forearm from perpendicular to the shoulder), the triceps brachii is the agonist, acting eccentrically.

One-Joint and Multi-Joint Muscles[2]

Muscle groups and individual muscles have layers. In the limbs the deepest layers are closest to the bones and the superficial layers are closer to the skin. In the torso, however, some of the deepest layers of muscle are deeper than the bones, and they are closest to the thoracic, abdominal, or pelvic cavities and organs.

Different muscles can cross different numbers of joints. Some can cross one joint, and some can cross two joints; some muscles in the hands and feet cross 8 or 9 joints, and some muscles in the spine cross

---

[2] While the terms *one-joint* and *multi-joint* are not used exclusively by Body–Mind Centering (BMC), the approach to muscular repatterning in BMC is the most sophisticated use of these concepts that I have encountered.

12 to 15 joints. The diaphragm has an effect on over 100 joints. It crosses some of those directly and affects others by way of fascial and skeletal connections.

With a few exceptions, the deeper the layer of muscle or muscle tissue, the shorter it is.[3] The shortest, deepest layers of muscle that cross one joint are called monoarticular, or one-joint muscles. These one-joint muscles have very specific actions and support articulation and discrimination at each joint. They are essential for the integrity and alignment of individual joints.

As the muscle layers get more and more superficial, they become longer and broader, and they cross more joints. If a muscle crosses more than one joint, every time it acts it has a direct effect on all of the joints it crosses as well as an indirect effect on all of the joints in the body. These longer muscles are called multi-joint muscles if they cross two or more joints. The multi-joint muscles connect all the parts of the limbs together, and they integrate the limbs into the torso. They give us the ability to negotiate large shifts of weight and movement of the whole body through space, or, in the diaphragm, to coordinate sophisticated shape changes in the torso.

Every joint has both one-joint and multi-joint muscles that surround it. Every joint has the possibility of discrete and specific movement, and the potential for being integrated into a flow of movement that travels through the whole body.

When we forget that we have the potential to move with specificity and articulation in every joint, we might never find some of the movement possibilities that are available to us. When we only use bigger and more superficial muscles, we work too hard. On the other hand, when we focus only on the deep one-joint muscles, we can forget to look at the whole picture of movement. All the layers are essential for healthy and efficient joint movement.

Kinetic Chains of Muscles

In addition to examining specific muscles around a single joint or the layers of muscles from deep to superficial, we can also consider how the muscles work together in kinetic chains.[4] In this case we no longer consider individual muscles but the ways that they are linked together by connective tissue into long chains of dynamic action.

Whenever we engage a single muscle, it has an effect on the rest of the body by way of the connective tissue. From anywhere in the body, movement follows a kinetic chain from one muscle to another through the direct relationships of the connective tissues that link the individual muscles and through the sensory-motor pathways of the nervous system that sequence the firing of the muscles.

Never in life do we use a single muscle to do a task. In an efficient, integrated movement, we engage enough muscles to get sufficient power for the task without expending too much energy or recruiting so many muscles that we get in our own way.

FUNDAMENTAL PRINCIPLES OF SKELETAL MUSCLES

The following are basic ideas on how muscles work in relationship to the bones and nerves. Understanding these principles can help to cultivate an awareness of the complexity and sophistication of the muscular system. Also, this awareness might prevent the oversimplifying that is so limiting to our movement choices.

---

[3] Exceptions are as follows: the extensor digitorum brevis in both the hands and feet, which lies on top of the extensor digitorum longus, and the psoas minor in the torso, which runs along the surface of the psoas major. Also, the psoas major and the diaphragm are some of the deepest muscles in the body, and both cross many joints.

[4] I first encountered the term *kinetic chains* in my study of Laban Movement Analysis and the Bartenieff Fundamentals, though it is used by a variety of therapeutic modalities.

An enormous difference also exists between the weight traveling clearly through the bones and the weight passively hanging in the joints. In this case, when we hang in a joint, the ligaments around that joint must negotiate the weight, and the weight doesn't translate clearly from bone to bone.

Bones support weight; muscles move bones. There is an enormous difference between how the muscles work when they are moving the bones into place to take weight and how they work when they are actually attempting to hold the weight themselves.

When the muscles take on a weight-bearing function, they overwork and become rigid and fixed. If the bones bear weight instead, the muscles can stay constantly moving and continuously make micro-adjustments to create efficient movement and dynamic stillness rather than disconnection and locking in the joints.

Muscles work best when they can calibrate tone. The basic definition of the word *tone* is readiness to respond. A tissue that has high tone needs less stimulation before a response is elicited because the tissue is more prepared to respond. On the other hand, a tissue with a lower tone needs more stimulation before a response happens.

Although it is related, this is not the same thing as sensitivity. A tissue can be very sensitive and have low tone. It might register a stimulus at a very fine level but not react until it receives a great deal of that stimulus. Alternatively, a tissue can have high tone and low sensitivity, where it is very ready to respond but not actually responding because it isn't picking up any stimulus.

All tissues need to be able to change tone in response to changes in the environment, both internal and external. The important thing is not the absolute state of tone but the tissue's ability to adapt.

If the tone of a muscle or group of muscles is too low, when a muscle is needed to participate in a task it might not be readily available and other muscles must compensate. This can lead to imbalances in the joint space, ligament sprains, and muscle strains.

On the other hand, if a muscle or group of muscles is too high in tone, the muscle tissue burns more energy than is necessary, is more likely to overwork, and creates imbalances in the joint space that lead to injury.

Because the muscles have a rich supply of nerve endings, they are able to calibrate their tone to a very sophisticated degree. This means that they can be incredibly efficient about using just enough effort to get the job done.

Muscles calibrate tone and cultivate awareness through negotiating resistance. The nervous system receptors in the muscle tissue are called spindles, a specialized kind of proprioceptor, or self-sensor. One of the things that they sense is what happens in the muscles when they meet resistance. These proprioceptive spindles then use that information to set the level of tone for the muscles so that each muscle can meet or match the resistance it encounters.

Muscles build tone by meeting greater and greater amounts of resistance. Resistance is an essential source of feedback for the proprioceptors and is based on sensing the relationship between the muscle tissue and the source of resistance (often gravity). When a muscle has the opportunity to engage with many different degrees of resistance, it learns to adapt and calibrate its level of tone.

When there is no resistance, the nerve endings in the muscles get no feedback, and the muscles don't have the ability to use the nerves to sense changes in tone or to make finely tuned adjustments to the muscle tone.[5]

---

[5] The nervous system is not the only way that we get information about the body. Cells are able to communicate with each other directly and through the fluid systems of the body; juxtacrine, paracrine, and endocrine signaling are examples of this.

Muscles pull. In a concentric contraction, the pulling power of the muscle is greater than the resistance. In an eccentric contraction, the pulling power of the muscle is less than the resistance. In an isometric contraction, the pulling power of the muscle is exactly the same as the resistance.

In all of these cases the muscle is firing and the molecules in the myofibrils are ratcheting together to pull. The muscle is never actively pushing the fibers in a way that slides them apart—that happens because the resistance is greater than the pulling force being generated.

So, how is it that we can push something away? Any joint movement includes a part that is lengthening and a part that is shortening. Whether or not the joint is flexing, extending, or rotating, some muscles are lengthening and some are shortening. The shortening muscles are concentrically contracting; the lengthening muscles are in various degrees of relaxation or are eccentrically contracting.

Flexibility and strength are about the relationship between the nervous system and the muscles. A classic definition of flexibility is the ability of the muscle to lengthen, and a classic definition of strength is the ability of the muscle to generate force and speed. Both flexibility and strength in the muscles are functions of the nervous system as much as they are functions of the ability of the muscle fibers and connective tissues to adapt in length.

In the vast majority of situations, flexibility is not determined by the actual physical length of the muscle or of the muscle fibers that compose that muscle. The resting length of the muscle, its tone, and the amount it will lengthen are all set by the proprioceptive nerve endings in the muscle. This setting is established in the nervous system through previous experiences regarding what is appropriate, safe, and functional.

The amount of strength a muscle has is more dependent on its physical properties, including the actual number of muscle fibers. Muscle strength is also a product of the way that the nervous system recruits fibers and organizes the surrounding muscles and kinetic chains. When the nervous system is inefficient in the way it recruits and organizes muscles, it diminishes the functional strength of a muscle by creating a situation where the muscle has to exert effort to overcome resistance from other muscles in the body.

Increasing flexibility and strength is a process of reeducating the nervous system through conscious attention and practice as much as it is about stretching and repetitions.

CONCLUSION

Muscles surround joints and wrap around bones in incredibly sophisticated spiraling layers. Embryologically, muscles follow fluid pathways from the center of the body out into the limbs. The three-dimensionality of the pathways of the muscles allows them to have incredibly nuanced effects on the bones that they move.

In a three-dimensional paradigm, it is clear that for each individual, the muscles weave together into unique patterns of dynamic lengthening and shortening that create the movements of daily life, such as walking and talking, opening a bottle, or brushing teeth. What creates integrated movement for one person is not the same pattern that creates integrated movement for another.

When traditional ideas about muscles shape our movement choices, we end up with faulty generalizations and assumptions about the role of muscles in creating movement and support.

What happens when we expect that in any given situation every person will use his or her muscles in the same way? That there is a "correct" sequence of muscle actions to perform a movement? That this way works for every person? And, that working harder makes a person stronger?

When we assume that we can generate a final and complete analysis of the unique and complex sequences of muscular action that are expressed in each person's movement choices, we create obstacles and limit the ways that new choices can arise. If we instead observe with a mind open to possibilities, examining each person's pattern becomes an opportunity to witness the incredible variety of ways that we can successfully execute the simplest actions.

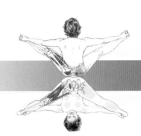

CHAPTER 5

INSIDE THE ASANAS

An asana, or yoga pose, is a container for an experience. An asana is not an exercise for strengthening or stretching a particular muscle or muscle group, although it might have that effect.

It is a form that we inhabit for a moment, a shape that we move into and out of, a place where we might choose to pause in the continuously flowing movement of life. In yoga poses, we experience a cross section of a never-ending progression of movement and breath, extending infinitely forward and backward in time.

Each asana is a whole-body practice where we can witness how things arise, how they are sustained, and how they dissolve or are transformed. We can see how we are affected by the experience of moving into the pose, being in the pose, and moving out of the pose, and how that might affect other places in our lives where we meet change. As long as we are in the matrix of space and time, we are never actually still.[1]

While we might choose different aspects of a pose to focus on, the asana itself is a composite of all the possible points of focus, and the whole experience is greater than the sum of its parts.

WHAT IS ASANA ANALYSIS?

How, then, can we possibly analyze the anatomy of an asana? Because we believe asana is more of a process than a final product, in the creation of this text it was a challenge to decide which moments to photograph and which parts of the anatomy to focus on.

For the purposes of this book, we tried to find the moments that capture the most recognizable parts of common asanas and analyzed them from the perspective of the musculoskeletal system and the breathing mechanism. We could just as well have chosen to focus on the organs or the endocrine system or the connective tissue and found something equally fascinating to discuss in every asana.

In each asana we chose a starting position and then determined the skeletal joint actions and muscular joint actions that could give rise to the asana.

STARTING POSITIONS AND THE BASE OF SUPPORT

In the first years of life, a baby learns fundamental movement skills: how to use different bases of support, how to negotiate a relationship to gravity, and how to move through space.

The base of support is the parts of the body that are on the ground and through which the weight-bearing forces are transmitted down to the earth, resulting in some supporting energy generated upward into the body. When we change our base of support, we change our experience of ourselves in relationship to gravity and space.

The feet—supporting the legs and pelvis—have evolved specifically to accomplish this for adult humans. The lessons you learn from standing on the earth can be applied to any other base of support you may experience. This is perhaps why simple standing poses are considered a starting point for asana practice by many yoga traditions.

---

[1] "Each bodily movement is embedded in a chain of infinite happenings from which we distinguish only the immediate preceding steps and, occasionally, those which immediately follow" (Laban 1966, p. 54).

The poses in this book are arranged by a starting position that is determined by the base of support. Any asana can arise from a variety of starting positions; we have tried to use the simplest entry points for each pose:

Standing—Supported on the soles of the feet (page 71)

Sitting—Supported on the base of the pelvis (page 125)

Kneeling—Supported on the knees, shins, and tops of the feet (page 163)

Supine—Supported on the back surface of the body (page 181)

Prone—Supported on the front surface of the body (page 211)

Arm support—Supported on the upper limbs (page 223)

SKELETAL JOINT ANALYSIS

After identifying the base of support for the asana, we analyze movement in the skeletal joints, asking the following questions:

In the axial skeleton

What is the spine doing?

Is it maintaining a shape and moving through space, or is it actually articulating?

If the spine is articulating, what is the joint action?

If the spine is not articulating and is moving through space, what is actually articulating?

In the appendicular skeleton

What joint is the focal joint (the point of focus)?

Is the focal joint articulating or moving through space, or both?

If the focal joint is articulating, what is the joint action?

If the focal joint is moving through space, what is actually articulating?

Please note, because the images are moments isolated from the full phrase of movement, there is no way to know the sequence in which the movements were made. The order in which things are listed is not any indication of what sequence is best, appropriate, or most effective. There is no single correct way to get into or out of these poses, and each choice you make will give rise to a different experience.

MUSCULAR SYSTEM ANALYSIS

Once it is clear what the main joint actions are, then we can consider the muscles. This is a more complex process because we have to take into account the relationship to gravity and other major points of resistance to determine which muscles to include as possibly being involved.

To narrow down the muscles to focus on, we ask the following questions:

In articulating joints

What is the joint action? What causes the joint action?

Is it going with gravity so that the weight of the body or the limbs creates the joint action? (If so, we're looking for eccentric muscle actions to modulate the pull of gravity.)

Does the joint action involve lifting the weight of the body or the limbs away from the floor, or moving against another kind of resistance? (If this is the case, we're looking for concentric muscle actions to overcome the pull of gravity.)

In joints that aren't articulating but are instead maintaining a position or neutral alignment

Are there outside forces, such as the pull of gravity or the action of another body part, that would pull the joint away from that alignment if nothing were active? (If so, then even though there is not a change in the joint, changing muscle actions may be necessary to maintain the alignment as it moves through space.)

An understandable question that could arise at this point is: Since the poses are all static, why wouldn't all the muscles just be doing isometric contractions?

We are describing how to come into the pose from a starting position, rather than how to be in the pose. Even if you maintain a pose for a period of time, the muscle actions that got you there from the starting point are likely still present.

The idea that we are ever not in movement is an illusion, one of the veils of maya (a Sanskrit word for the temporary truths that arise from the world of matter). On the most fundamental level, the actions of the breathing structures never cease. We might talk about a final position, but in fact the image we hold is a kind of snapshot in a never-ending progression of movement, extending infinitely forward and backward in time. As long as we are alive, we are never actually still.

INFORMATION FOR EACH POSE

With an occasional variation, each pose description includes the following sections:

Name—Each asana is presented with its Sanskrit name and its translated English name. Additionally, some descriptive text is added to clarify the meaning or context of the pose's name.

Classification—Poses are classified by their symmetry, base of support, and general action (forward bending, twisting, balancing, etc.).

Skeletal joint actions—The main joints that are involved in the process of moving into the asana are identified according to their actions (flexion, extension, adduction, abduction, rotation, etc.).

Muscular joint actions—Muscles that create the joint actions are identified by the kind of contraction (concentric, eccentric, or isometric), their name, and their general actions.

Notes—From a certain perspective, yoga is the practice of uncovering and resolving obstructions in the human system. Practicing yoga asanas is a systematic way of illuminating those obstacles and learning from them. Presented are the most common opportunities for observing potential obstacles and suggestions for deepening your exploration.

Breathing—Specific shape-changing challenges to the respiratory mechanism are outlined.

DRAWINGS

The asana images in this book are based on photographs of various models that were taken during several sessions (figure 5.1). Some of the perspectives are quite unusual because they were shot from below using a large acrylic sheet or from above using a ladder.

The photos were used as reference for the anatomical illustrator, who posed her skeleton in the various positions and sketched the bones by hand. After a round of corrections, the muscles and other structures were added using computer software, and several more rounds of corrections and adjustments were made to produce the final images.

The labeling of the structures in each drawing, as well as the various arrows and other indicators, were added last. Muscles are sometimes labeled in the drawings for reference purposes and may not be active in that particular asana. If you find a muscle in the text that is not labeled on the accompanying drawing, use the muscle index on page 270 to find an illustration of that muscle.

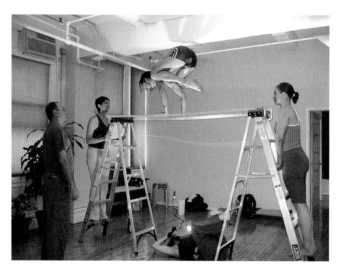

Figure 5.1   *Yoga Anatomy* photo shoot at The Breathing Project in New York City. Leslie Kaminoff (far left) supervises as the photographer, Lydia Mann, shoots Derek's bakasana from below the acrylic sheet. Janet and Elizabeth stabilize the ladders. The final artwork from the resulting photo is on page 232.

CONCLUSION

It was often a challenge to know what to say about the actions in the joints and muscles for each asana. Each body is unique. Each body has different ways of responding to gravity, different pathways for recruiting muscles, and a different amount of tone in the joint capsules and ligaments. Two people can use different muscles to create the same joint action and then have completely different sensations of the experience in the same asana. We each have our own way to distinguish between sensations of stretching and lengthening, working and holding, or pain and release.

In a few cases we list muscles that are lengthening but are not necessarily active—described as *passively lengthening*—to distinguish them from muscles that are actively lengthening in an eccentric contraction. For some people these muscles will have the sensation of stretching, but for others there will not be a sensation of stretching until far past an appropriate range of motion. For still others these muscles might actually be so easy to lengthen that they would do better to engage in an eccentric contraction and modulate the range of motion.

Our choices about how to move through an asana will depend on our starting condition. For example, if I have very open shoulders, then I might think about internally rotating the humerus relative to the scapula, while my neighbor with less mobility in the glenohumeral joint is rolling the arms open as much as she can. Both actions could be functional in adho mukha svanasana (downward-facing dog pose) because the point of the asana (on a body level) is not to do it right, but to find the relationship between all the parts of the body that will let the experience of the asana resonate throughout the whole body—cells, tissues, fluids, and systems.

The ways we initiate a movement, whether from the bones and muscles or from the endocrine system or the blood, have a tremendous impact on the quality of the movement. With practice and skillful observation we can see from the initiation how the movement will travel through the body and the effect it will have on the body systems. An understanding of what we are activating to move into an asana will help us understand the nature of the asana and the effect it has on the skeletal, muscular, nervous, and endocrine systems; the mind; and the spirit.

The asana is not just the final arrangement of the limbs and spine, but is the full process of coming into that arrangement. If we look at the process rather than the final product, we are able to develop variations that increase or decrease the challenge of the asana without feeling that we aren't actually doing the asana until we get our head to our knee, our hands to the floor, or some other concrete goal. We are able to adapt the asana to the individual so that each person can find a unique embodiment of the asana.

Because yoga practice is fundamentally experiential, the information in this book is intended to be an inspiration to explore your own body. Perhaps you will understand more clearly something you've experienced as a result of reviewing this material. On the other hand, some anatomic detail may capture your interest and move you to investigate it through a pose that is being depicted. In either case, this book will have served its purpose if it supports you in these explorations.

Please take these ideas as a launching point for discussion and exploration, rather than as the final word on how to achieve the pose. And then, once you've found your own way in, try it the opposite way!

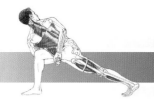

CHAPTER 6

STANDING POSES

When you stand, you bear weight on the only structures in the body that have specifically evolved to hold you up in the uniquely human stance—the feet. The architecture of the feet, along with their musculature, shows nature's unmatched ability to reconcile and neutralize opposing forces.

These amazing structures are massively over-engineered for the way most people use them in the civilized world. Stiff shoes and paved surfaces teach our feet to be passive and inarticulate. Fortunately, yoga exercises are usually done barefoot, with much attention given to restoring the strength and flexibility of the foot and lower leg.

In a yoga practice, early lessons frequently center on the simple act of standing upright—something humans do from the time they are about a year old. If you can feel your weight releasing into the three points of contact between the foot and the earth, you may be able to feel the support that the earth gives back to you through the action of the arches of the foot and the muscles that control them.

Release and support, giving and receiving, and inhaling and exhaling—these are all ways of translating *sthira sukham asanam*, Patañjali's fundamental description of asana in chapter 2 of the *Yoga Sutras*. T.K.V. Desikachar's translation sums it up well when he defines *sthira* as "alertness without tension" and *sukha* as "relaxation without dullness" (*The Heart of Yoga*, II.46). The fundamental lessons you learn from standing postures can illuminate the practice of other asanas.

Standing positions have the highest center of gravity of all the starting points, and the effort of stabilizing that center makes standing poses by definition brhmana (see chapter 1, page 20).

Tadasana

Mountain Pose

tah-DAHS-anna

tada = mountain

The name of this pose evokes many images that relate to a stable, rooted base of support and a crown that reaches for the heavens.

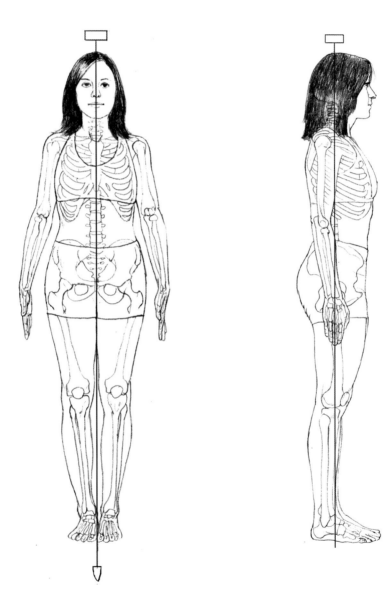

Classification

Symmetrical standing pose

Skeletal joint actions		
Spine	**Upper limbs**	**Lower limbs**
Neutral extension or mild axial extension	Neutral extension, forearm pronation	Hip adduction and neutral extension, knee neutral extension, ankle dorsiflexion

Notes

A wide variety of muscles in the torso engage in a combination of concentric and eccentric contractions to maintain the curves of the spine in relationship to the pull of gravity. In each person a different combination of flexors and extensors will be active in varying kinds and degrees of contractions to maintain the postural support needed.

The arches of the feet are engaged and connecting with the support of the pelvic floor, lower abdomen, rib cage, cervical spine, and crown of the head.

Nothing lasting can be built on a shaky foundation. This may be why tadasana is considered by many yoga traditions to be the starting point of asana practice. It is interesting that this pose is almost identical to the anatomical position—the starting reference point for the study of movement and anatomy. The only major difference between the two positions is that in tadasana, the forearms are pronated (the palms of the hands are facing the sides of the thighs rather than forward).

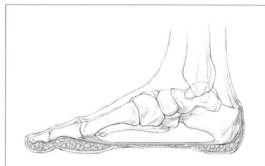

Nonmuscular support and padding for the foot: the fat pads (yellow) and plantar fascia (blue). The muscles of the foot occupy the space between the plantar fascia and the bones.

This body position is also uniquely human, because humans are the only true biped mammals on the planet. Humans are also the least stable of creatures, possessing the smallest base of support, the highest center of gravity, and (proportionately) the heaviest brain balancing atop it all.

The base of support of this pose—the feet—offers a beautiful image of how the forces of yielding and support operate in the human system. The essential structure of the foot can be represented by a triangle. The three points of the triangle are the three places where the foot's structure will rest on a supporting surface: the heel, the distal end of the first metatarsal, and the distal end of the fifth metatarsal. The lines connecting these points represent three of the arches, lines of lift through which postural support is derived: the medial longitudinal arch, the lateral longitudinal arch, and the transverse (metatarsal) arch. There is also a fourth arch, called the medial transverse arch or the tarsal arch, that is across the tarsal bones from the navicular to the cuboid.

(continued)

From underneath, the two triangles of the feet can be joined to show the size and shape of the base of support for tadasana. The plumb line that passes through the body's center of gravity in this position should also fall through the exact center of this base.

The many layers of musculature (see the top figure on page 75) all combine to create lift, balance, and movement of the 28 bones (26 major bones and 2 sesamoid bones) of the foot, which has evolved to be an incredibly adaptable structure able to move you smoothly over uneven terrain.

The foot has evolved over millions of years in a world with no roads or sidewalks. When the adaptability of the foot is no longer needed during locomotion, the deeper muscles that support the arches can weaken, eventually leaving only the superficial, nonmuscular plantar fascia responsible for preventing the collapse of the foot. The stress this places on the plantar fascia frequently leads to plantar fasciitis and heel spurs.

The practice of standing postures in general, and tadasana in particular, is one of the best ways to restore the natural vitality, strength, and adaptability of the feet. Once your foundation is improved, it is much easier to put the rest of your house in order.

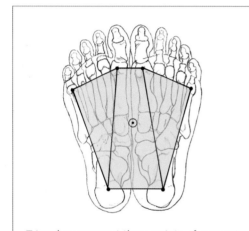

Triangles represent three points of support of each foot.

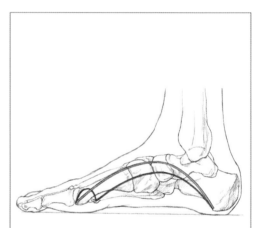

Three of the arches of the foot.

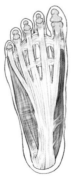

The plantar fascia, the most superficial layer of support for the foot. The more the arch support muscles weaken, the more pressure is put on the plantar fascia, which can result in plantar fasciitis and heel spurs.

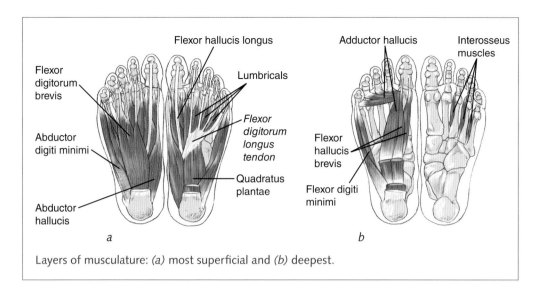

Flexor hallucis longus

Flexor digitorum brevis

Lumbricals

Flexor digitorum longus tendon

Abductor digiti minimi

Flexor digitorum longus tendon

Abductor hallucis

Quadratus plantae

Adductor hallucis

Interosseus muscles

Flexor hallucis brevis

Flexor digiti minimi

a

b

Layers of musculature: *(a)* most superficial and *(b)* deepest.

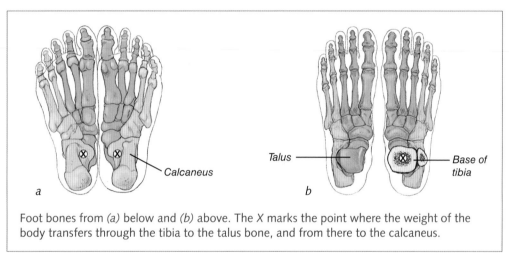

Calcaneus

a

Talus

Base of tibia

b

Foot bones from *(a)* below and *(b)* above. The X marks the point where the weight of the body transfers through the tibia to the talus bone, and from there to the calcaneus.

Breathing

Tadasana is an excellent position for observing the interaction between the muscles that are used for postural support and the muscles that create shape change in the abdominal and thoracic cavities. When there is clear support from the feet, legs, and spine, there is more mobility in the rib cage and shoulder girdle to allow for the movement of the breath.

(continued)

Tadasana Variation

Samasthiti

Equal Standing, Prayer Pose

sama = same, equal; *sthiti* = to establish, to stand

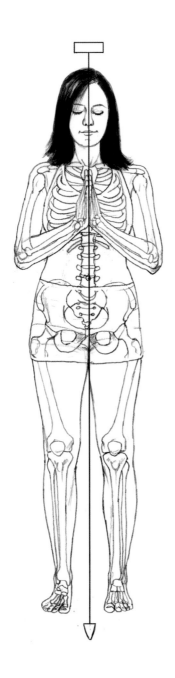
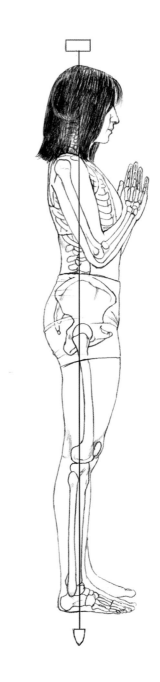

Notes

Samasthiti has a wider base than tadasana because the feet are placed with the heels under the sitting bones (or wider) rather than as close to each other as possible. All the standing poses that are executed from this base, as opposed to tadasana, consequently have a wider, more stable base of support.

Additionally, the head is lowered and the hands are in namaste (prayer) position. This is typical of the starting point of a sun salutation, a vinyasa, which is used by many systems of hatha yoga to connect asanas into a flowing sequence.

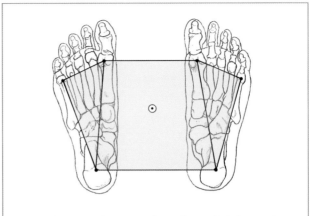

Base of support for samasthiti. The circled dot marks where the center line of gravity falls.

Terminology Note

In the Ashtanga tradition of Sri K. Pattabhi Jois, the term *samasthiti* refers to what is here described as *tadasana*. In the teaching tradition of Sri T. Krishnamacharya and his son, T.K.V. Desikachar, the term *tadasana* refers to a standing pose with the arms overhead, and balancing on the balls of the feet (the base of which is depicted below).

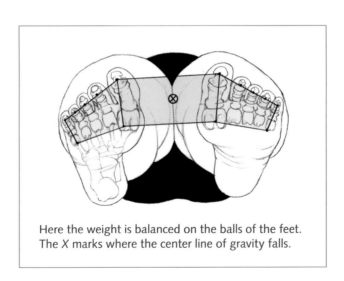

Here the weight is balanced on the balls of the feet. The X marks where the center line of gravity falls.

Utkatasana

Chair Pose, Awkward Pose

OOT-kah-TAHS-anna

utkata = awkward

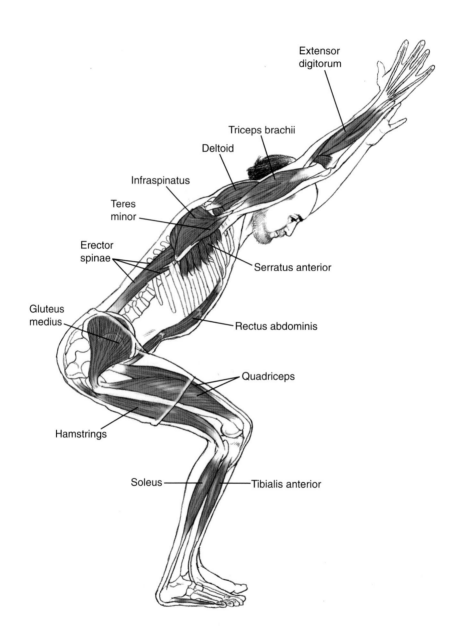

Extensor
digitorum

Triceps brachii

Deltoid

Infraspinatus

Teres
minor

Erector
spinae

Serratus anterior

Gluteus
medius

Rectus abdominis

Quadriceps

Hamstrings

Soleus

Tibialis anterior

Classification

Symmetrical standing pose

Skeletal joint actions

Spine	Upper limbs	Lower limbs
Axial extension	Scapular upward rotation, abduction, and elevation; shoulder flexion; elbow extension	Hip flexion, knee flexion, ankle dorsiflexion

Muscular joint actions

Spine

Concentric contraction

To maintain alignment of spine:	**To prevent anterior tilt of pelvis and over-extension of lumbar spine:**
Intertransversarii, interspinalis, transverso-spinalis, erector spinae	Psoas minor, abdominal muscles

Upper limbs

Concentric contraction

To upwardly rotate, abduct, and elevate scapula:	**To extend elbow:**
Upper trapezius, serratus anterior	Anconeus, triceps brachii
To stabilize and flex shoulder joint:	
Rotator cuff, coracobrachialis, pectoralis major and minor, anterior deltoid, biceps brachii (short head)	

Lower limbs

Concentric contraction	*Eccentric contraction*
To resist tendency to widen knee (abduct at hip):	**To allow hip and knee flexion and ankle dorsiflexion without collapsing into gravity:**
Gracilis, adductor longus and brevis	Gluteus maximus, medius, and minimus; hamstrings at hip joint; vastii; soleus; intrinsic muscles of foot

Notes

Shortness in the latissimus dorsi will interfere with lifting the arms overhead.

Overly arching the lumbar spine or overly flexing the hips can happen because of a collapse into gravity. Using the hamstrings to draw the ischial tuberosities (sitz bones) forward or using the psoas minor to lift the pubic bone can prevent tipping the pelvis too far forward without necessarily affecting the alignment of the spine.

The knees are very mobile in this position because they are partly flexed.

Gravity, rather than muscles working against each other, should be the main source of resistance in the pose. This is an interesting pose to explore a balance between effort and release.

Breathing

Maintaining axial extension (which minimizes breathing shape change) while engaging the largest, most oxygen-hungry muscles of the body presents a challenge that requires efficiency of effort and breath.

Uttanasana

Standing Forward Bend

OOT-tan-AHS-anna

ut = intense; *tan* = stretch

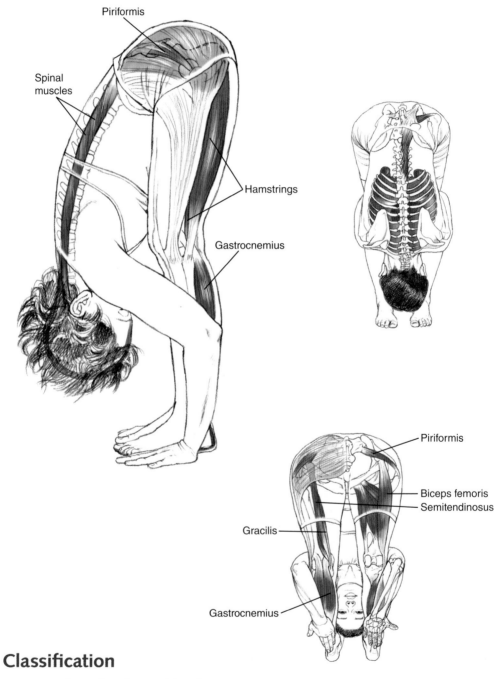

Classification

Symmetrical standing forward-bending pose

Skeletal joint actions		
Spine	**Lower limbs**	
Mild flexion	Hip flexion, knee extension	

Muscular joint actions		
Spine		
Passively lengthening		
Spinal muscles		
Lower limbs		
Concentric contraction	*Eccentric contraction*	*Passively lengthening*
To maintain knee extension: Articularis genu, vastii	**To maintain balance:** Intrinsic and extrinsic muscles of foot and lower leg	Hamstrings, gluteus medius and minimus (posterior fibers), gluteus maximus, piriformis, adductor magnus, soleus, gastrocnemius

Notes

The less the hips can flex in this pose, the more spinal flexion occurs.

Tightness in the hamstrings, spinal muscles, and gluteals reveals places where there is excess effort. In this pose, gravity should do the work of moving one deeper into the pose. People experiencing tightness in the back of the legs sometimes pull themselves down by using the muscles of hip flexion, which creates tightness and congestion in the front of the hip joints. A more efficient choice would be to release the knees, find some softness in the hip joints, and allow the spine to release. After the spine has released, extending the legs can produce an even lengthening along the entire back line of the body.

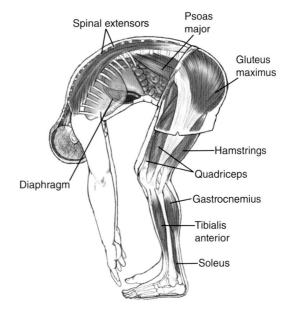

If the hamstrings are tight, slightly bending the knees helps release the spine.

Breathing

Deep hip flexion and spinal flexion compress the abdomen and restrict the ability of the abdomen to move with the breath. This compression combined with gravity also moves the center of the diaphragm cranially, so more freedom is needed in the back of the rib cage for the breath.

Utthita Hasta Padangusthasana

Extended Hand–Toe Pose

oo-TEE-tah HA-sta pad-an-goosh-TAHS-anna

utthita = extended; *hasta* = hand; *pada* = foot; *angusta* = big toe

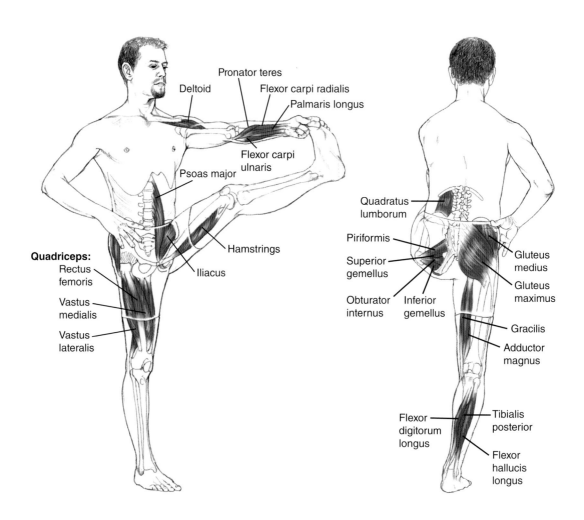

Classification

Asymmetrical standing balancing pose

Skeletal joint actions

Spine	Upper limbs	Lower limbs	
	Lifted arm	**Standing leg**	**Lifted leg**
Neutral spine, level pelvis	Shoulder flexion and slight adduction, elbow extension, finger flexion	Neutral hip extension, neutral knee extension	Hip flexion and slight adduction to midline, neutral knee extension, neutral ankle dorsiflexion

Muscular joint actions

Spine

To calibrate concentric and eccentric contractions to maintain neutral alignment of spine: Spinal extensors and flexors	*Concentric contraction*
	To counter rotation in torso from pull of arm: Rotatores, transversospinalis, external and internal oblique

Upper limbs

Lifted arm

Concentric contraction

To stabilize, flex, and slightly adduct shoulder joint: Rotator cuff, coracobrachialis, pectoralis minor, anterior deltoid, biceps brachii (short head)	**To grasp big toe:** Flexors of hand and fingers

Lower limbs

Standing leg		**Lifted leg**	
Concentric contraction	*Eccentric contraction*	*Concentric contraction*	*Passively lengthening*
To keep knee in neutral extension and balance on single leg: Articularis genu, quadriceps, hamstrings, intrinsic and extrinsic muscles of foot and lower leg	**To allow lateral shift of pelvis over standing foot for balance and to keep pelvis level:** Gluteus medius and minimus, piriformis, superior and inferior gemellus, tensor fasciae latae	**To flex hip and slightly adduct leg toward midline:** Psoas major, iliacus, rectus femoris, pectineus, adductor brevis and longus	Gluteus maximus, hamstrings, gastrocnemius, soleus

(continued)

Notes

Tightness in the hamstrings or gluteus maximus in the lifted leg can cause spinal flexion by pulling on the pelvis and tipping it posteriorly. This can lead to hip extension or knee flexion in the standing leg. It is better to bend the knee in the lifted leg and find neutral curves in the spine, neutral extension in the standing hip, and knee extension (but not hyperextension) in the standing leg. Weakness in the hip flexors (psoas major, iliacus, and rectus femoris) of the lifted leg can also cause the quadratus lumborum to attempt to help with lifting the leg.

Abductors of the standing leg are working eccentrically; if they are weak or tight, the hip of the lifted leg hikes up or the rotators (gluteus maximus, piriformis, and obturators) try to stabilize the pelvis and the pelvis rotates on the standing leg, rather than staying level and facing forward.

The more strength and adaptability you have in the feet and ankles, the more options you have for finding balance on the standing leg.

Breathing

In maintaining this balancing pose, if there isn't enough support in the deep hip flexors (psoas major and iliacus), the stabilizing action in the abdominal muscles combines with the bracing action of the arms, which can create an overall reduction of breathing capacity. If excessive muscular tension exists, the reduced volume of breath is not sufficient to fuel the effort, and the movement caused by increasing the volume of breath might compromise the balance.

Utthita Hasta Padangusthasana Variation

With Spine Flexed

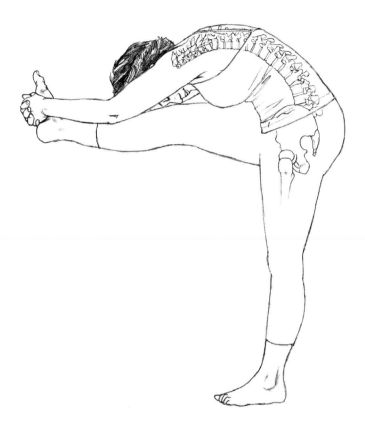

Notes

In this variation on utthita hasta padangusthasana, the lifted leg is parallel to the floor and the head comes to the knee. Because the individual lowers the head to the knee instead of lifting the leg to the head, the balance is much more challenging. For those who are accustomed to going to their extreme range of motion, this pose is a valuable exploration of precision in placement.

There is less length required in the hamstrings but much more mobility required in the muscles of the back. For the spine to flex so deeply, the spinal muscles must lengthen a great deal while the abdomen softens. This is an excellent pose for exploring how the conventional holding patterns in the abdomen can be released and finding balance from the support of the pelvic floor rather than engaging abdominals and muscles of the lower back and posterior rib cage.

Vrksasana

Tree Pose

vrik-SHAHS-anna

vrksa = tree

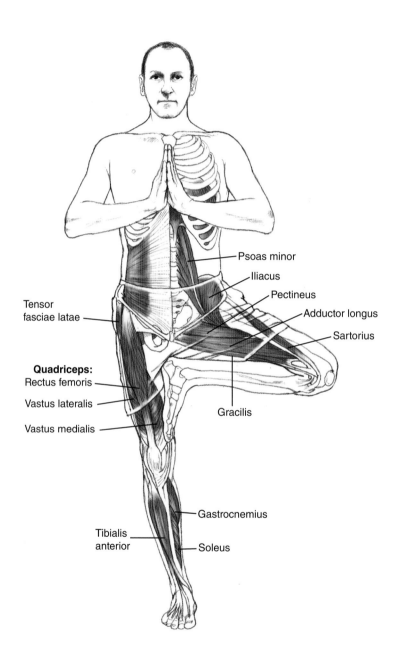

Psoas minor

Iliacus

Pectineus

Tensor
fasciae latae

Adductor longus

Sartorius

Quadriceps:
Rectus femoris

Vastus lateralis

Vastus medialis

Gracilis

Gastrocnemius

Tibialis
anterior

Soleus

Classification

Asymmetrical standing balancing pose

Skeletal joint actions

Spine	Upper limbs	Lower limbs	
		Standing leg	**Lifted leg**
Neutral spine, level pelvis	Slight shoulder flexion and adduction; elbow flexion; forearm pronation; wrist, hand, and finger extension	Neutral hip extension, neutral knee extension	Hip flexion, external rotation, and abduction; knee flexion; ankle dorsiflexion

Muscular joint actions

Spine

To calibrate concentric and eccentric contractions to maintain neutral alignment of spine:
Spinal extensors and flexors

Lower limbs

Standing leg		Lifted leg	
Concentric contraction	*Eccentric contraction*	*Concentric contraction*	*Passively lengthening*
To keep knee in neutral extension and balance on single leg: Articularis genu, quadriceps, hamstrings, intrinsic and extrinsic muscles of foot and lower leg	**To allow lateral shift of pelvis over standing foot for balance and to keep pelvis level:** Gluteus medius and minimus, piriformis, obturator internus, superior and inferior gemellus, tensor fasciae latae	**To flex hip:** Iliacus, psoas major **To externally rotate leg and open it to side:** Gluteus maximus, gluteus medius and minimus (posterior fibers), piriformis, obturator internus and externus, superior and inferior gemellus, quadratus femoris **To press foot into standing leg:** Adductor magnus and minimus	Pectineus, adductor longus and brevis, gracilis

(continued)

Notes

As in the previous pose, abductors on the standing leg are working eccentrically; if they are weak or tight, the hip of the lifted leg hikes up or the rotators (gluteus maximus, piriformis, and obturators) try to stabilize the pelvis and the pelvis rotates on the standing leg, rather than staying level and facing forward.

The more strength and adaptability you have in the feet and ankles, the more options you have for finding balance on the standing leg.

The action of the lifted leg, where the knee is drawn up and out to the side, is actually a very complex movement muscularly: Hip flexors are active to lift the knee, but with external rotation and abduction, hip extension also becomes involved. Then, in order to press the foot into the standing leg while keeping the knee out to the side (and without tipping the pelvis forward), the hip joint needs to adduct without flexion. Of course, the higher on the standing leg the foot is, the less it is necessary to press the foot in because the weight of the leg holds the foot in place. However, if it is necessary to use the adductors to press the foot into the standing leg, it is important to find adductors that are more posterior, such as the adductor magnus. Anterior adductors, such as the pectineus (which is short and active on many of us, in part from sitting so much), will tip the pelvis forward and internally rotate the lifted leg at the same time they are trying to adduct.

Breathing

Compared to the variation of vrksasana (page 89) with the arms elevated or utthita hasta padangusthasana (page 82), the upper body is freer to participate in respiratory movements in this pose.

Vrksasana Variation

With Arms Elevated

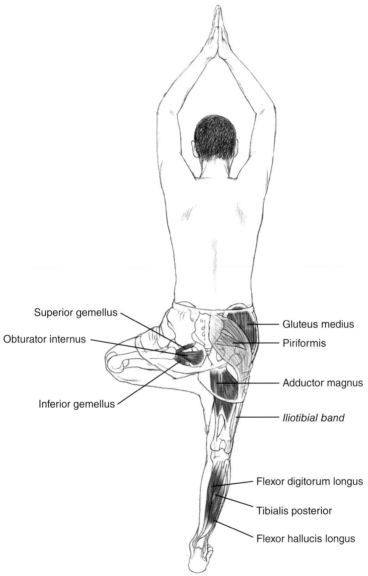

Superior gemellus

Obturator internus

Inferior gemellus

Gluteus medius

Piriformis

Adductor magnus

Iliotibial band

Flexor digitorum longus

Tibialis posterior

Flexor hallucis longus

Notes

This variation creates a higher center of gravity by placing the arms overhead and is therefore a more challenging balance for some. On the other hand, for other people, having the arms extended makes the balance easier.

Breathing

Because of the stabilizing action of the muscles that keep the arms overhead, the thoracic movements of the breath might encounter more resistance in this position. In addition, the higher center of gravity tends to produce a stronger stabilizing action in the abdominal muscles. Taken together, these factors combine to reduce the overall excursion of the diaphragm.

Garudasana

Eagle Pose

gah-rue-DAHS-anna

garuda = a fierce bird of prey; the vehicle (vahana) of the Hindu god Vishnu, usually described as an eagle but sometimes as a hawk or kite

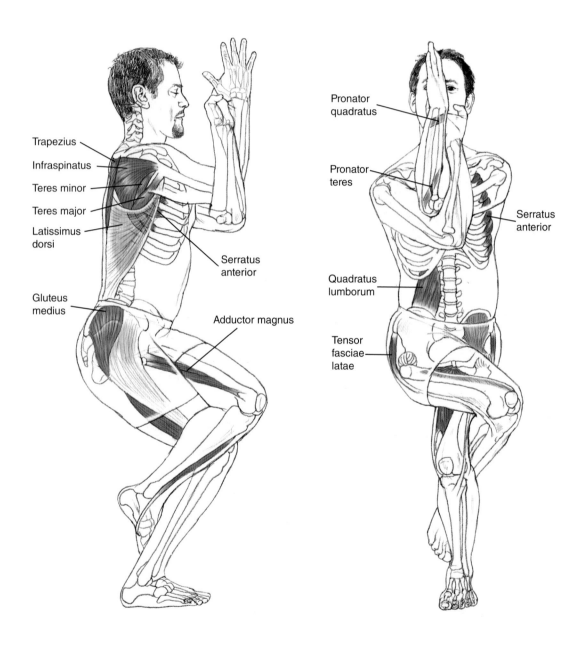

Classification

Asymmetrical standing balancing pose

Skeletal joint actions

Spine	Upper limbs	Lower limbs
Neutral spine or flexion	Scapular abduction and upward rotation, shoulder flexion and adduction, elbow flexion, forearm pronation	Hip flexion, internal rotation, and adduction; knee flexion and internal rotation (of tibia); ankle dorsiflexion; lifted foot pronation

Muscular joint actions

Spine

To calibrate concentric and eccentric contractions to maintain neutral alignment of spine:

Spinal extensors and flexors

Upper limbs

Concentric contraction	Passively lengthening
To abduct and upwardly rotate scapula:	Rhomboids, middle and lower trapezius, latissimus dorsi
Serratus anterior	
To stabilize, flex, and adduct shoulder joint:	
Rotator cuff, coracobrachialis, pectoralis major and minor, anterior deltoid, biceps brachii (short head)	
To flex elbow:	
Biceps brachii, brachialis	
To pronate forearm:	
Pronator quadratus and teres	

Lower limbs

Standing leg		Lifted leg	
Concentric contraction	Eccentric contraction	Concentric contraction	Passively lengthening
To adduct and inwardly rotate hip:	**To allow hip and knee flexion and ankle dorsiflexion without collapsing into gravity:**	**To flex, adduct, and internally rotate hip:**	Gluteus maximus, gluteus medius and minimus (posterior fibers), piriformis, obturator internus, superior and inferior gemellus
Pectineus, adductor brevis and longus	Gluteus maximus, medius, and minimus; hamstrings at hip joint; vastii; soleus; intrinsic muscles of foot	Psoas major, iliacus, pectineus, adductor brevis and longus, gracilis	
	To allow lateral shift of pelvis over standing foot and to maintain balance by actively lengthening:	**To flex and internally rotate knee:**	
	Gluteus medius and minimus, piriformis, obturator internus, superior and inferior gemellus	Popliteus, gracilis, medial hamstrings	
		To pronate foot:	
		Peroneals, extensor digitorum longus	

(continued)

Notes

To achieve the full entwining of the legs, the standing leg needs to flex at the hip and knee as well as the lifted leg.

This position of hip flexion with internal rotation and adduction is not structurally easy (the shape of the hip socket generally makes it easier to externally rotate when the hip is flexed). The action of adduction with internal rotation especially lengthens the piriformis, obturator internus, and superior and inferior gemellus. Restriction along the outside of the thigh can also come from shortness in the muscles that attach near the top of the iliotibial (IT) band: The gluteus maximus and tensor fasciae latae attach directly to the IT band, and the gluteus medius and minimus attach nearby and affect it strongly.

This position can be challenging for the knees: If the hips don't perform the actions of adduction and internal rotation, the knees are forced to compensate and possibly overrotate. Paying attention to internally rotating the tibia can help prevent this overmobilization of the knee.

This action in the legs is generally stabilizing for the sacroiliac (SI) joint because it encourages the pelvic halves to move together in the front, which can bring congruence to the edges of the SI joint on the anterior surfaces of the sacrum and ilium.

Breathing

The scapulae need to be able to both abduct and rotate upwardly. If the scapulae are pulled down too much, the movement of the rib cage is unnecessarily inhibited.

From the standpoint of shape, center of gravity, and breathing, this is the most compacted of the one-legged balancing postures. The entwining of the arms compresses the front of the rib cage, and freedom to move in the posterior portion of the rib cage is essential.

Natarajasana

King of the Dancers Pose

not-ah-raj-AHS-anna

nata = dancer; *raja* = king

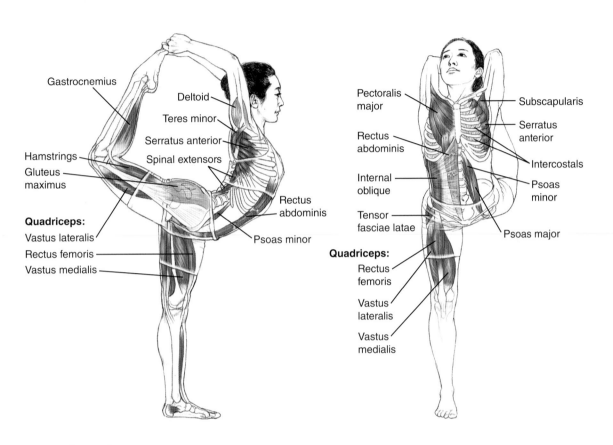

Classification

Asymmetrical standing backward-bending balancing pose

Skeletal joint actions			
Spine	**Upper limbs**	**Lower limbs**	
		Standing leg	**Lifted leg**
Extension	Scapular upward rotation, abduction, and elevation; shoulder flexion, adduction, and external rotation; forearm supination; hand and finger flexion	Hip flexion, neutral knee extension	Hip extension and slight adduction to midline, knee flexion, ankle plantar flexion

(continued)

Muscular joint actions

Spine

Concentric contraction	*Eccentric contraction*
To extend spine: Spinal extensors	**To prevent hyperextension at lumbar spine:** Psoas minor, abdominal muscles

Upper limbs

Concentric contraction	*Passively lengthening*
To abduct, upwardly rotate, and elevate scapula: Serratus anterior, upper trapezius **To stabilize, flex, and adduct shoulder joint:** Rotator cuff, coracobrachialis, pectoralis major (upper fibers), anterior deltoid, biceps brachii (short head) **To rotate forearm and grasp foot:** Supinator and flexors of hand and fingers	Rhomboids, latissimus dorsi, pectoralis major (lower fibers), pectoralis minor

Lower limbs

Standing leg		Lifted leg	
Concentric contraction	*Eccentric contraction*	*Concentric contraction*	*Passively lengthening*
To keep knee in neutral extension and balance on single leg: Articularis genu, quadriceps, hamstrings; intrinsic and extrinsic muscles of foot and lower leg	**To allow lateral shift:** Gluteus medius and minimus, piriformis, obturator internus, superior and inferior gemellus, tensor fasciae latae **To allow anterior tilt of pelvis without falling forward:** Hamstrings, gluteus maximus	**To create hip extension and knee flexion to enter pose:** Hamstrings **To create hip extension, internal rotation, and adduction:** Adductor magnus **To create hip extension:** Gluteus maximus **To extend knee and increase hip extension against resistance of hand grasping foot:** Vastii	Iliacus, psoas major, rectus femoris

Notes

Scapular mobility is important in this full-arm version, both for getting the arms into position without overmobilizing the shoulder joints and for mobility in the extension of the thoracic spine.

Using the latissimus dorsi to accomplish spinal extension interferes with the range of motion of the scapulae and restricts the movement of the rib cage.

It can be a challenge to keep the lifted leg adducted and internally rotated at the hip joint in this asana. Although you might find more extension through external rotation at the hip joint, this involves the risk of overmobilizing the SI joint or overextending the lumbar spine.

As in dhanurasana (page 216), the additional resistance created by the hands grasping the foot can put pressure in vulnerable spots such as the knee and lower back.

Breathing

In this pose the excursion of the diaphragm is minimized by the deep spinal extension. The more clearly support is found in the intrinsic muscles of the spine and the less effort needed in the superficial muscles of the back and torso, the more movement is available for the breath.

Virabhadrasana I

Warrior I

veer-ah-bah-DRAHS-anna

Virabhadra = the name of a fierce mythical warrior

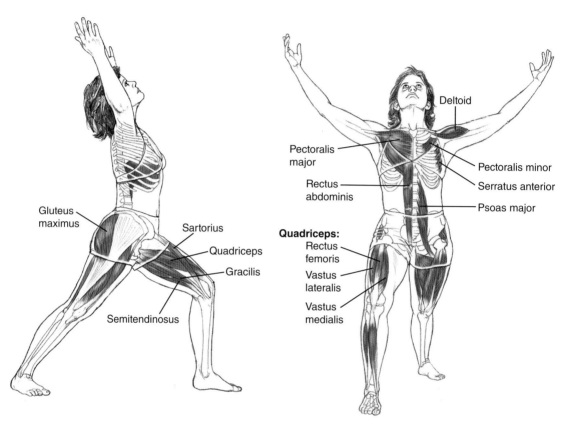

Classification

Asymmetrical standing backward-bending balancing pose

Skeletal joint actions			
Spine	**Upper limbs**	**Lower limbs**	
		Front leg	**Back leg**
Extension, slight rotation for chest to face forward, pelvis level	Scapular abduction and upward rotation, shoulder abduction and external rotation, slight elbow flexion, forearm supination	SI joint nutation, hip flexion, knee flexion, ankle dorsiflexion	SI joint counternutation, hip extension and adduction, knee extension, ankle dorsiflexion and foot supination at heel and pronation at forefoot

Muscular joint actions

Spine

Concentric contraction	Eccentric contraction
To extend spine:	**To prevent hyperextension at lumbar spine:**
Spinal extensors	Psoas minor, abdominal muscles
To rotate chest forward:	**To support weight of head as neck extends:**
Internal oblique (front leg side); external oblique (back leg side)	Rectus capitis, longus capitis and colli, verticalis, scalenes

Upper limbs

Concentric contraction	
To abduct and upwardly rotate scapula:	**To stabilize and abduct shoulder joint:**
Serratus anterior	Rotator cuff, biceps brachii (long head), middle deltoid
To supinate forearm:	
Supinator	

Lower limbs

Front leg		Back leg	
Concentric contraction	Eccentric contraction	Concentric contraction	Eccentric contraction
To resist tendency to widen knee (abduct at hip):	**To allow hip and knee flexion and ankle dorsiflexion without collapsing into gravity:**	**To extend hip:**	**To allow outer ankle to lengthen without collapsing inner knee or inner foot:**
Gracilis, adductor longus and brevis	Gluteus maximus, hamstrings at hip joint, vastii, soleus, intrinsic and extrinsic muscles of foot	Hamstrings at hip joint, gluteus medius (posterior fibers), adductor magnus, gluteus maximus	Peroneals
	To level and center pelvis over feet and to maintain balance side to side (the narrower the stance, the more active and long these muscles need to be):	**To extend knee:**	
		Articularis genu, vastii	
	Gluteus medius and minimus; piriformis, superior and inferior gemellus	**To maintain arches of foot without inhibiting dorsiflexion of ankle:**	
		Intrinsic muscles of foot	

(continued)

Notes

In warrior I, warrior II (page 100), and other lunging poses, the weight of the body (in relationship to gravity) creates the flexion at the knee and hip of the front leg—the muscles of the front leg are eccentrically contracting, which means they are active as they lengthen to keep from moving too far into flexion.

The abductors in the front leg also need to be active eccentrically to level and orient the pelvis to the front leg and to maintain balance. If they shorten they can pull the front knee too far to the side or twist the pelvis out of alignment.

In general, muscles become fatigued more quickly when they are close to their maximum working length, so it can take some time to build stamina in these positions.

Many different things are said about the amount of external or internal rotation of the back leg in warrior I. What is consistently true is that the back leg is extended and to some degree adducted (in comparison to warrior II, where the back leg is extended and abducted).

We suggest that the back leg be organized from the spiral of the foot upward, and that the bones of the foreleg, thigh, and pelvis orient themselves to create a clear pathway from foot to spine. If the back leg is organized in this way, the amount of internal or external rotation in the hip joint varies from person to person, but the joint spaces can be balanced and the back leg is a strong support for the weight of the torso. This also takes some of the effort of this position from the front leg.

In the back foot, the subtalar joint and the joints between the tarsals and metatarsals need to articulate so that the back part of the foot supinates so the calcaneus can clearly connect to the floor and the forefoot pronates so the toes can clearly connect to the floor. If the foot doesn't articulate in this way, the outer ankle can be overmobilized and weakened.

The amount of rotation needed in the spine depends on how articulate the SI joints and hip joints are—the less mobile the lower limbs are, the more rotation is needed in the spine to orient the chest forward.

Breathing

The lower body needs to be both articulate and strong to provide enough support (sthira) for the breath to move freely in the upper body (sukha). The various challenges of the lunging position in these warrior poses create interesting parameters for exploring the breath mechanics.

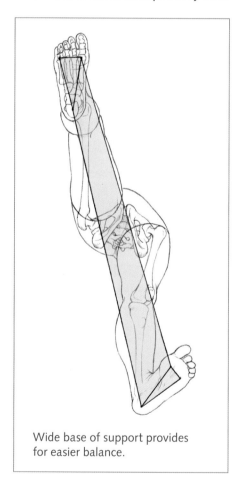

Wide base of support provides for easier balance.

Virabhadrasana I Variation

With Longer Stance

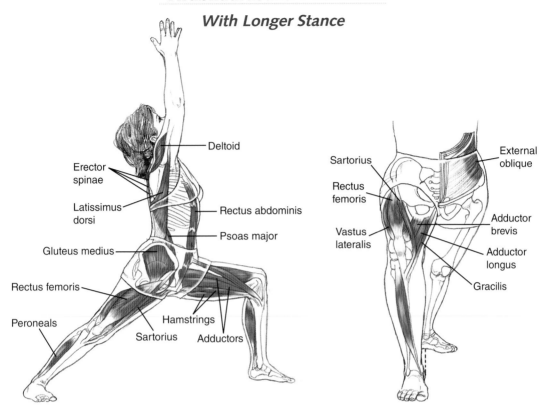

Deltoid

Erector spinae

Latissimus dorsi

Gluteus medius

Rectus femoris

Peroneals

Hamstrings

Sartorius

Adductors

Rectus abdominis

Psoas major

Sartorius

Rectus femoris

Vastus lateralis

External oblique

Adductor brevis

Adductor longus

Gracilis

Notes

Different arrangements of the feet affect where you experience the challenges of this pose. The shorter stance (from front to back) requires less mobility in the pelvis, so the support of the legs might feel more accessible. The width of the base makes the balance easier, but the higher center of gravity in the shorter pose might actually make the balance feel more precarious for some.

In a longer, narrower stance it may be easier to balance because the center of gravity is lower. However, it may also be harder to balance because the stance is narrower and the adductors then have to be effective at a greater length. The extended stance also requires more mobility in the SI joints, hips, knees, ankles, and feet, and requires the muscles that resist flexion in the hips and knees to work at a greater length, which can make the pose feel less stable.

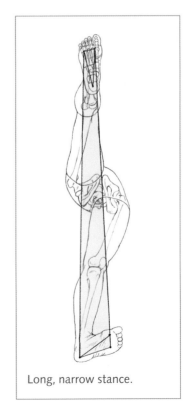

Long, narrow stance.

Virabhadrasana II

Warrior II

veer-ah-bah-DRAHS-anna

Virabhadra = the name of a fierce mythical warrior

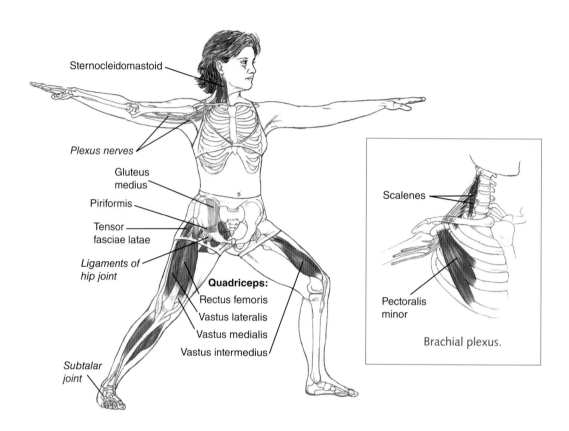

Sternocleidomastoid

Plexus nerves

Gluteus medius

Piriformis

Tensor fasciae latae

Ligaments of hip joint

Quadriceps:
Rectus femoris
Vastus lateralis
Vastus medialis
Vastus intermedius

Subtalar joint

Scalenes

Pectoralis minor

Brachial plexus.

Classification

Asymmetrical standing pose

Skeletal joint actions			
Spine	**Upper limbs**	**Lower limbs**	
		Front leg	**Back leg**
Neutral spine, slight rotation for chest to orient to side, head rotated to face front leg, pelvis level	Scapular abduction, shoulder abduction and external rotation, forearm pronation	SI joint nutation, hip flexion and abduction, knee flexion, ankle dorsiflexion	SI joint counternutation, hip extension and abduction, knee extension, ankle dorsiflexion, foot supination at heel and pronation at forefoot

Muscular joint actions

Spine

Alternating concentric and eccentric contractions	Concentric contraction
To maintain neutral alignment of spine: Spinal extensors and flexors	**To rotate chest to side:** External oblique (front leg side); internal oblique (back leg side)
	To rotate head toward front leg: Rectus capitis posterior, obliquus capitis inferior, longus capitis and colli, splenius capitis (front leg side); sternocleidomastoid, upper trapezius (back leg side)

Upper limbs

Concentric contraction	Passively lengthening
To abduct scapula: Serratus anterior	Pectoralis major and minor (particularly in back arm)
To stabilize and abduct shoulder joint: Rotator cuff, biceps brachii (long head), deltoid	
To pronate forearm: Pronator quadratus and teres	

Lower limbs

Front leg		Back leg	
Concentric contraction	Eccentric contraction	Concentric contraction	Eccentric contraction
To abduct hip: Gluteus medius and minimus	**To abduct hip and allow hip flexion without collapsing into gravity:** Gluteus maximus, piriformis, obturator externus, superior and inferior gemellus	**To extend and abduct hip:** Gluteus medius and minimus, hamstrings at hip joint, piriformis, obturator externus, superior and inferior gemellus	**To support inner knee:** Gracilis
	To allow hip and knee flexion and ankle dorsiflexion without collapsing into gravity: Hamstrings at hip joint, vastii, soleus, intrinsic and extrinsic muscles of foot	**To extend knee:** Articularis genu, vastii	**To allow outer ankle to lengthen without collapsing inner knee or inner foot:** Peroneals
		To maintain arches of foot without inhibiting dorsiflexion of ankle: Intrinsic muscles of foot	

(continued)

Notes

As in warrior I (page 96), the action of flexion in the front hip and knee is eccentric in relationship to the pull of gravity. Unlike warrior I, however, the abductors of the front leg are working concentrically to abduct the hip—because the foot is on the ground, this action is proximal and has the effect of rotating the pelvis open to the side.

In the back leg, simultaneous hip extension and abduction are challenging—the articulation of the pelvis and sacrum at the SI joint can take some of the pressure of these actions away from the ligaments and capsule of the hip joint.

Like warrior I, a wide variety of opinions exists about how much external rotation is needed in the back hip joint. The amount of rotation depends on a variety of factors and should arise from the action of the foot and whole leg, rather than being an isolated hip joint action.

The more mobility there is in the SI joint and hip joint of the front leg, the less spinal rotation is needed to turn the chest to face the side.

If the chest is not clearly facing sideways, the spreading of the arms can put pressure on the brachial plexus (the web of nerves that extend into the arm), which travels from the side of the cervical spine under the clavicle and under the pectoralis minor. Keeping the arms in line with the sides of the torso helps to prevent this compression, which can result in sensations of numbness or tingling in the arms.

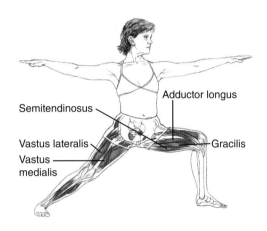

Virabhadrasana II with longer stance.

Breathing

In all the warrior poses the lower body needs to be both articulate and strong to allow the breath to move freely. In virabhadrasana II there may be more ease in the movement of the breath because there is less twist in the pelvis and spine than in virabhadrasana I. For some people this leg position is less effortful, which creates more ease in the breath as well.

Virabhadrasana III

Warrior III

veer-ah-bah-DRAHS-anna

Virabhadra = the name of a fierce mythical warrior

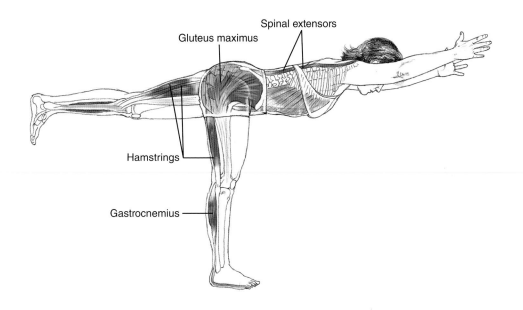

Classification

Asymmetrical standing balancing pose

Skeletal joint actions			
Spine	**Upper limbs**	**Lower limbs**	
		Standing leg	**Lifted leg**
Neutral spine or axial extension	Scapular upward rotation, abduction, and elevation; shoulder abduction; elbow extension	SI joint nutation, hip flexion and adduction, knee extension, ankle dorsiflexion	SI joint counternutation, neutral hip extension and rotation, knee extension, ankle dorsiflexion

(continued)

Muscular joint actions

Spine

Concentric contraction

To maintain alignment of spine:	To prevent anterior tilt of pelvis and overextension of lumbar spine:
Intertransversarii, interspinalis, transversospinalis, erector spinae	Psoas minor, abdominal muscles

Upper limbs

Concentric contraction

To upwardly rotate, abduct, and elevate scapula:	To extend elbow:
Upper trapezius, serratus anterior	Anconeus, triceps brachii
To stabilize and flex shoulder joint:	
Rotator cuff, coracobrachialis, pectoralis major and minor, middle deltoid, biceps brachii (short head)	

Lower limbs

Standing leg		Lifted leg
Concentric contraction	*Eccentric contraction*	*Concentric contraction*
To keep knee in neutral extension and balance on single leg:	**To control hip flexion:** Hamstrings	**To maintain neutral hip extension and rotation:**
Articularis genu, quadriceps, intrinsic and extrinsic muscles of foot and lower leg	**To allow lateral shift of pelvis over standing foot for balance and to keep pelvis level:** Gluteus medius and minimus, piriformis, superior and inferior gemellus	Hamstrings, adductor magnus, gluteus maximus

Notes

Keeping the pelvis level in this action requires the standing leg abductors to lengthen while they are active—gravity draws the unsupported side of the pelvis toward the floor. If the abductors instead shorten, they tilt the pelvis so that the opposite hip lifts away from the floor.

It can also be challenging to keep the lifted leg parallel, and using muscles that are extensors and internal rotators such as the medial hamstrings and adductor magnus balance the action of the gluteus maximus, which is both a powerful hip extensor and an external rotator.

Breathing

Much like in utkatasana (page 78), the combined actions of this pose (especially with the arms overhead) can engage some of the larger muscle groups of the torso. If the most superficial layers of muscle in the back (such as the latissimus dorsi) are used to maintain spinal alignment, they can inhibit the movement of the rib cage and make breathing even more challenging. It is better to work more efficiently in the deeper muscles of the spine.

Utthita Parsvakonasana

Extended Side Angle Pose

oo-TEE-tah parsh-vah-cone-AHS-anna

utthita = extended; *parsva* = side, flank; *kona* = angle

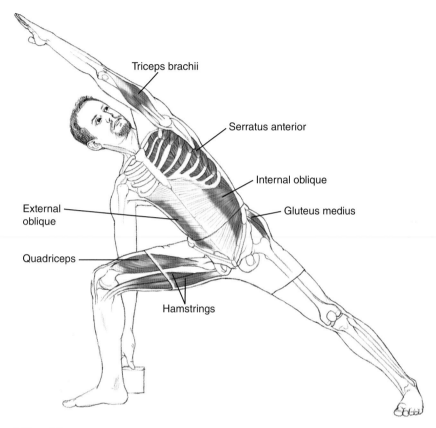

Triceps brachii

Serratus anterior

Internal oblique

External oblique

Gluteus medius

Quadriceps

Hamstrings

Classification

Asymmetrical standing pose

Skeletal joint actions				
Spine	**Upper limbs**		**Lower limbs**	
	Upper arm	**Lower arm**	**Front leg**	**Back leg**
Neutral spine or slight lateral flexion, slight rotation for chest to orient to side, head rotated to face upper arm	Scapular upward rotation, abduction, and elevation; shoulder abduction and external rotation; elbow extension; forearm pronation	Shoulder abduction, forearm pronation, wrist dorsiflexion	SI joint nutation, hip flexion and abduction, knee flexion, ankle dorsiflexion	S-I joint counter-nutation, hip extension and abduction, knee extension, ankle dorsiflexion, foot supination at heel and pronation at forefoot

(continued)

Muscular joint actions

Spine

Concentric contraction	Eccentric contraction
To rotate chest to side:	**To resist side bending into gravity:**
Internal oblique (back leg side); external oblique (front leg side)	Quadratus lumborum, latissimus dorsi, spinal muscles (back leg side)
To rotate head toward ceiling:	
Rectus capitis posterior, obliquus capitis inferior, longus capitis and colli, splenius capitis (back leg side); sternocleidomastoid, upper trapezius (front leg side)	

Upper limbs

Upper arm

Concentric contraction	Eccentric contraction
To upwardly rotate, abduct, and elevate scapula:	**To extend arm to overhead without falling into gravity:**
Serratus anterior	Rotator cuff, teres major, latissimus dorsi
To extend elbow:	
Triceps brachii, anconeus	

Lower limbs

Front leg		Back leg	
Concentric contraction	Eccentric contraction	Concentric contraction	Eccentric contraction
To abduct hip:	**To allow hip and knee flexion and ankle dorsiflexion without collapsing into gravity:**	**To extend and abduct hip:**	**To support inner knee:**
Gluteus medius and minimus, piriformis, obturator externus, superior and inferior gemellus	Gluteus maximus, hamstrings at hip joint, vastii, soleus, intrinsic and extrinsic muscles of foot	Gluteus medius and minimus, hamstrings at hip joint, piriformis, obturator externus, superior and inferior gemellus	Gracilis
		To extend knee:	**To allow outer ankle to lengthen without collapsing inner knee or inner foot:**
		Articularis genu, vastii	Peroneals
		To maintain arches of foot without inhibiting dorsiflexion of ankle:	
		Intrinsic muscles of foot	

Notes

The legs in this pose are performing the same actions as in warrior II (page 100), and similar muscle groups are active. In this pose, however, the weight of the torso falls more over the front leg, and the muscles of the front leg need additional strength, length, and stamina.

While the position of the upper arm alongside the head is similar to that of the arms in utkatasana (page 78) and virabhadrasana III (page 103), different muscles are required to maintain the arm position in this pose because of the different relationship to gravity. The action is also more eccentric than concentric, again because of the relationship of the weight of the arm to gravity.

Breathing

Even though the upper side of the breathing mechanism receives a strong lengthening action in this shape, the more interesting effect may be on the lower side of the body, where the dome of the diaphragm is driven cranially by the force of gravity acting on the abdominal organs. Breath action in this position provides very useful asymmetrical stimulation to the diaphragm and all the organs attaching to it.

Parivrtta Baddha Parsvakonasana
Revolved Side Angle Pose

par-ee-VRIT-tah BAH-dah parsh-vah-cone-AHS-anna

parivrtta = twist, revolve; *baddha* = bound; *parsva* = side, flank; *kona* = angle

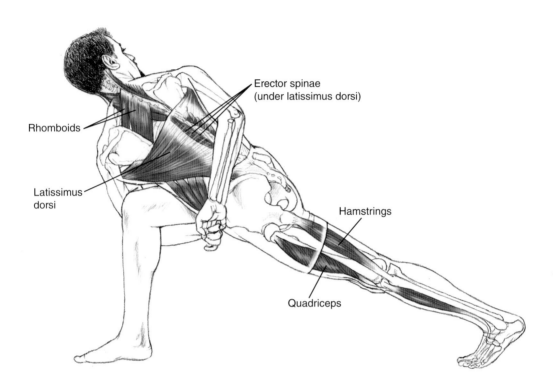

Erector spinae
(under latissimus dorsi)

Rhomboids

Latissimus dorsi

Hamstrings

Quadriceps

Classification

Asymmetrical standing twisting pose

Skeletal joint actions			
Spine	**Upper limbs**	**Lower limbs**	
		Front leg	**Back leg**
Axial rotation	Scapular downward rotation and abduction (moving toward adduction); shoulder internal rotation, extension, and adduction; elbow extension; forearm pronation; hand and finger flexion	SI joint nutation, hip flexion, knee flexion, ankle dorsiflexion	SI joint counternutation, hip extension and adduction, knee extension, ankle dorsiflexion, toe flexion

Muscular joint actions

Spine

Concentric contraction	Eccentric contraction
To rotate spine toward front leg: Erector spinae, internal oblique (front leg side); transversospinalis, rotatores, external oblique (back leg side) **To resist flexion caused by action of arms:** Spinal extensors	**To balance rotation around axis:** Transversospinalis, rotatores, external oblique (front leg side); erector spinae, internal oblique (back leg side)

Upper limbs

Concentric contraction	Eccentric contraction or passively lengthening
To stabilize humeral head: Rotator cuff **To internally rotate shoulder and prevent protraction:** Subscapularis, anterior deltoid **To extend arm back:** Teres major, posterior deltoid, latissimus dorsi **To extend shoulder and elbow:** Triceps brachii **To grasp:** Flexors of fingers and hand	Upper trapezius, pectoralis major and minor, serratus anterior, coracobrachialis

Lower limbs

Front leg		Back leg	
Concentric contraction	Eccentric contraction	Concentric contraction	Passively lengthening
To resist tendency to widen knee (abduct at hip): Gracilis, adductor longus and brevis	**To allow hip and knee flexion and ankle dorsiflexion without collapsing into gravity:** Gluteus maximus, hamstrings at hip joint, vastii, soleus, intrinsic and extrinsic muscles of foot **To level and center pelvis over feet and to maintain balance side to side (the narrower the stance, the more active and long these muscles need to be):** Gluteus medius and minimus, piriformis, superior and inferior gemellus	**To extend hip:** Hamstrings at hip joint, gluteus medius (posterior fibers), adductor magnus, gluteus maximus **To extend knee:** Articularis genu, vastii	Soleus, gastrocnemius

(continued)

Notes

In a spinal rotation around the axis of the spine (without side bending, flexing, or extending), note that the muscles that are concentrically contracting on one side of the body are eccentrically contracting on the opposite side. This ends up meaning that one layer of abdominals is concentrically contracting while the layer above or below is eccentrically contracting. This layering allows for a very finely tuned modulation of spinal actions and balance in the whole circumference of the torso.

Binding the arms in any position has a strong effect on the shoulder girdle and the spine. The anterior–inferior part of the glenohumeral joint capsule is the most vulnerable to dislocation. The binding of the arms in internal rotation and extension puts pressure on this part of the joint capsule, especially if the rest of the shoulder girdle is limited in its mobility. (This caution applies to binding in general because it allows for more leverage or force to be directed into the joint.)

In the process of coming into the bind, both the scapulae and arms abduct and then adduct. The adduction of the scapulae is usually the final step. If the scapulae have been depressed (pulled down the back) in addition to their other joint actions, their mobility is compromised.

Another compensation that happens if the shoulder girdle is restricted is spinal flexion. Flexion of the spine combined with rotation of the spine leaves the joints of the spine vulnerable to overmobilization. It is possible to use the leverage of the arms in their binding and against the leg to force the spine past an appropriate range of motion.

Breathing

The more open the pelvic structures are, the easier the balance and breathing is in this asana. Here, the upper body is firmly bound in rotation against the resistance of the lower body, so there is significant resistance to the movements of the diaphragm, abdomen, and rib cage.

Utthita Trikonasana

Extended Triangle Pose

oo-TEE-tah trik-cone-AHS-anna

utthita = extended; *tri* = three; *kona* = angle

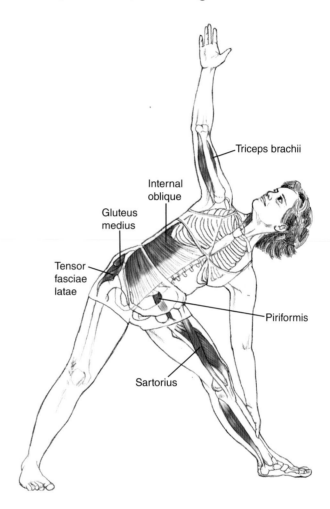

Triceps brachii

Internal oblique

Gluteus medius

Tensor fasciae latae

Piriformis

Sartorius

Classification

Asymmetrical standing pose

Skeletal joint actions			
Spine	**Upper limbs**	**Lower limbs**	
		Front leg	**Back leg**
Neutral spine, slight rotation for chest to orient to side, head rotated on axis to face upward	Scapular abduction, shoulder abduction and external rotation, neutral forearm	SI joint nutation, hip flexion and abduction, knee extension, slight ankle plantar flexion	SI joint counternutation, hip extension and adduction, knee extension, ankle dorsiflexion, foot supination at heel and pronation at forefoot

(continued)

Muscular joint actions

Spine

Alternating concentric and eccentric contractions	Concentric contraction	Eccentric contraction
To maintain neutral alignment of spine: Spinal extensors and flexors	**To rotate chest to side:** Internal oblique (back leg side); external oblique (front leg side) **To rotate head toward ceiling:** Rectus capitis posterior, obliquus capitis inferior, longus capitis and colli, splenius capitis (back leg side); sternocleidomastoid, upper trapezius (front leg side)	**To resist side bending into gravity:** Quadratus lumborum, latissimus dorsi, spinal muscles (back leg side)

Upper limbs

Concentric contraction

To abduct scapula:	To stabilize and abduct shoulder joint:
Serratus anterior	Rotator cuff, biceps brachii (long head), deltoid

Lower limbs

Front leg		Back leg	
Concentric contraction	Eccentric contraction	Concentric contraction	Eccentric contraction
To abduct hip: Gluteus medius and minimus **To extend knee:** Articularis genu, vastii	**To abduct hip and allow hip flexion without collapsing into gravity:** Gluteus maximus, piriformis, obturator externus, superior and inferior gemellus **To allow hip flexion without collapsing into gravity:** Hamstrings at hip joint **To maintain integrity of foot without collapsing:** Intrinsic and extrinsic muscles of foot	**To extend hip:** Hamstrings at hip joint **To extend knee:** Articularis genu, vastii **To support inner knee:** Gracilis **To maintain arches of foot without inhibiting dorsiflexion of ankle:** Intrinsic muscles of foot	**To maintain extension of hip while adducting:** Piriformis, obturator externus, superior and inferior gemellus **To allow hip to abduct:** Gluteus medius and minimus **To allow outer ankle to lengthen without collapsing inner knee or inner foot:** Peroneals

Notes

In utthita trikonasana, as in utthita parsvakonasana (page 105), the weight of the torso falls mostly over the front leg. Because the front knee is extended, the action in this pose is shifted from the eccentric contraction of the quadriceps to keep the knee from bending too deeply (as in utthita parsvakonasana) to the balance of actions around the joint that create a clear pathway of support without hyperextending the knee.

Pain or pressure in that front knee can be a result of lack of mobility in the hip joints and pelvis; whether the lack of movement is from short adductor muscles or another cause, the next place the movement can travel is the inner knee. Sensations from within the knee (or any joint) are important signals to stop what you're doing and adjust your action or position.

In the back leg, the muscles that cross the side of the pelvis, the outer hip, and the outer knee need to be actively lengthening (eccentrically contracting) to allow the pelvis to tilt sideways (adduct) over the leg. If these muscles cannot lengthen, the pelvis does not move as much, and the spine side bends. On the other hand, if these muscles are not active at all, the weight of the torso can collapse into gravity and put pressure in the outer hip joint or outer ankle joint.

Does the spine rotate in utthita trikonasana? There are many different ways utthita trikonasana is taught, and good reasons exist for each perspective. In general, the more articulated the SI joints, pelvic halves, and hip joints are, the less rotation is needed in the spine for the chest to face sideways. For example, if the front leg has a tight pectineus, which is an adductor, the pelvis may rotate to the floor, and the spine has to counterrotate more to open the chest. The rotation of the spine can accommodate a variety of obstacles in the legs. As in all the poses, maintaining balanced joint space is far more important than achieving a particular range of motion in one or two joints.

Utthita Trikonasana Variation

With Longer Stance

Notes

In some approaches to yoga, the feet are placed much farther apart than in other approaches. The variety of leg positions has an effect on which joints need more mobility and which muscles have to work at longer or shorter ranges.

When the feet are placed farther apart, the front leg muscles have to work at a greater length, but the muscles of the outer hip of the back leg work at a shorter length. It may actually be easier to keep the spine from side bending when the feet are farther apart. On the other hand, the pelvis may rotate toward the floor less when the feet are closer together.

There is no absolutely correct dis-

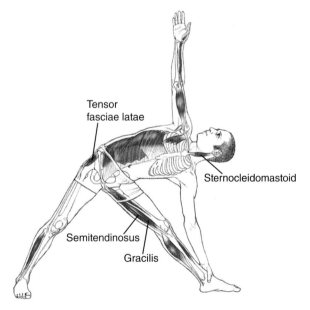

tance for placing the feet in utthita trikonasana; each distance provides different information about the relationship between the torso and the legs.

Parivrtta Trikonasana

Revolved Triangle Pose

par-ee-VRIT-tah trik-cone-AHS-anna

parivrtta = to turn around, revolve; *tri* = three; *kona* = angle

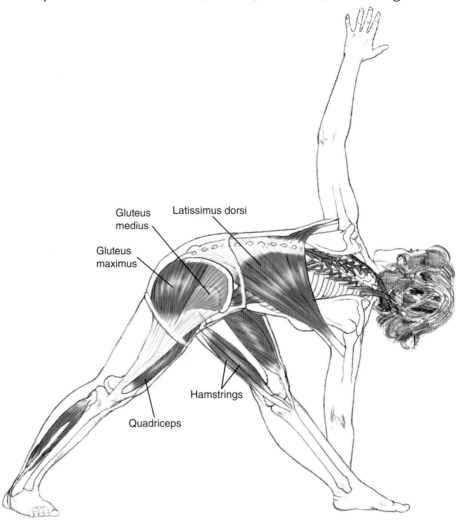

Gluteus medius

Latissimus dorsi

Gluteus maximus

Hamstrings

Quadriceps

Classification

Asymmetrical standing twisting pose

Skeletal joint actions			
Spine	**Upper limbs**	**Lower limbs**	
		Front leg	**Back leg**
Axial rotation	Scapular abduction, shoulder abduction and external rotation, neutral forearm	Hip flexion, knee extension, slight ankle plantar flexion	Mild hip flexion, knee extension, ankle dorsiflexion, foot supination at heel and pronation at forefoot

Muscular joint actions

Spine

Alternating concentric and eccentric contractions	Concentric contraction	Eccentric contraction
To maintain neutral alignment of spine: Spinal extensors and flexors	**To rotate spine toward front leg:** Erector spinae, internal oblique (front leg side); transversospinalis, rotatores, external oblique (back leg side)	**To balance rotation around axis:** Transversospinalis, rotatores, external oblique (front leg side); erector spinae, internal oblique (back leg side)

Upper limbs

Concentric contraction	
To abduct scapula: Serratus anterior	**To stabilize and abduct shoulder joint:** Rotator cuff, biceps brachii (long head), deltoid

Lower limbs

Front leg		Back leg		
Concentric contraction	Eccentric contraction	Concentric contraction	Eccentric contraction	Passively lengthening
To extend knee: Articularis genu, vastii	**To allow hip flexion:** Hamstrings at hip joint, gluteus maximus **To level and center pelvis over feet and to maintain balance side to side:** Gluteus medius and minimus, piriformis, superior and inferior gemellus, intrinsic and extrinsic muscles of foot	**To extend knee:** Articularis genu, vastii **To maintain arches of foot without inhibiting dorsiflexion of ankle:** Intrinsic muscles of foot	**To allow hip flexion without dropping back leg forward:** Hamstrings at hip joint, gluteus medius (posterior fibers), adductor magnus, gluteus maximus **To allow outer ankle to lengthen without collapsing inner knee or inner foot:** Peroneals	Soleus, gastrocnemius

(continued)

Notes

The rotation of the spine in this pose requires the muscles on the outsides of the hip joints to be very long, and because of the narrowness of the base, the same muscles are very actively modulating their actions to keep from falling side to side. This eccentric action of lengthening while stabilizing for balance can make this pose feel very precarious.

If the legs and pelvis do not have the mobility to flex and rotate as much as needed, the spine may flex to compensate. Rotating the spine when it is in a flexed position leaves the joints along the back of the spine vulnerable to overmobilizing. It is important in this pose to respect the range of motion available in the spine and to avoid using the pressure of the hand on the floor or against the leg to force movement.

Breathing

In parivrtta trikonasana, the more open the pelvic structures are, the easier the balance and breathing is. Otherwise, the upper body is held stiffly in rotation against the resistance of the lower body, and the diaphragm, abdomen, and rib cage encounter considerable resistance to their movements.

Parsvottanasana

Intense Side Stretch

parsh-voh-tahn-AHS-anna

parsva = side, flank; *ut* = intense; *tan* = to stretch

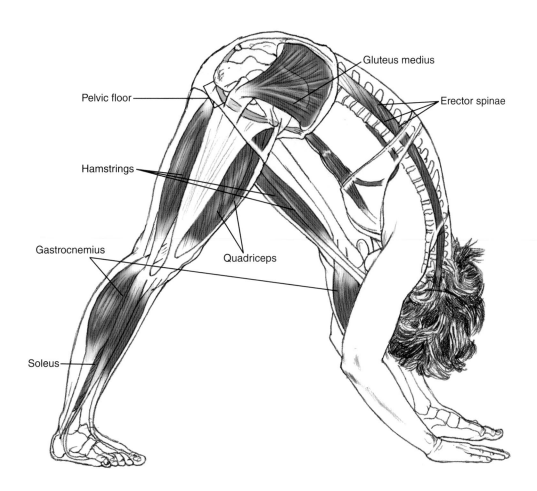

Classification

Asymmetrical standing forward-bending pose

	Skeletal joint actions	
Spine	**Lower limbs**	
	Front leg	**Back leg**
Mild flexion	Hip flexion, knee extension, slight ankle plantar flexion	Mild hip flexion, knee extension, ankle dorsiflexion, foot supination at heel and pronation at forefoot

(continued)

Muscular joint actions

Spine

Concentric contraction or passively lengthening

Erector spinae

Lower limbs

Front leg		Back leg		
Concentric contraction	*Eccentric contraction*	*Concentric contraction*	*Eccentric contraction*	*Passively lengthening*
To extend knee: Articularis genu, vastii	**To allow hip flexion:** Hamstrings at hip joint, gluteus maximus **To level and center pelvis over feet and to maintain balance side to side:** Gluteus medius and minimus, piriformis, superior and inferior gemellus, intrinsic and extrinsic muscles of foot	**To extend knee:** Articularis genu, vastii **To maintain arches of foot without inhibiting dorsiflexion of ankle:** Intrinsic muscles of foot	**To allow hip flexion without dropping back leg forward:** Hamstrings at hip joint, gluteus medius (posterior fibers), adductor magnus, gluteus maximus **To allow outer ankle to lengthen without collapsing inner knee or inner foot:** Peroneals	Soleus, gastrocnemius

Notes

The action of the legs in parsvottanasana is almost the same as in utthita trikonasana (page 111), and this asana can be a challenge to balance in for the same reason—the narrowness of the base and the need for the outer hip muscles to be both long and active. Additionally, if you are accustomed to using your eyes to help you balance, this position with the head rolled forward might be interesting.

   This forward-bending action is more intense in the hamstrings of the front leg than uttanasana because of the asymmetry of the pose: The back leg's position directs the flexion more specifically into the front leg hip joint, and mobility in the spine can compensate less for lack of mobility in the leg. (This is seen in an even more extreme form in hanumanasana [page 156].)

Parsvottanasana Variation

With Arms in Reverse Namaskar

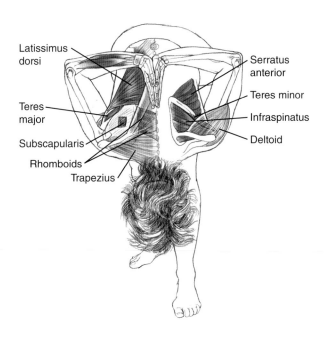

Notes

This arm position can be incorporated into a variety of asanas. It requires a fair amount of mobility in the shoulder girdle, and if the scapulae are not able to move easily on the rib cage, bringing the hands into this position may direct excessive pressure into the shoulder joints themselves.

Bringing the arms into the position generally involves abducting the scapulae and spreading them away from the spine before the final actions of adducting the scapulae and moving them toward the spine. This final movement of adduction is much more challenging if the spine is flexed or if the scapulae are depressed and pulled down the back.

(continued)

Parsvottanasana Variation
With Spine Flexed

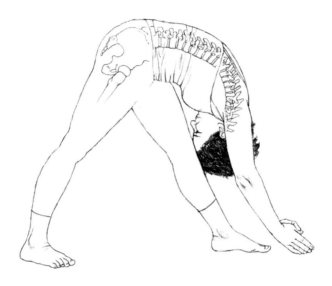

Notes

In this variation on parsvottanasana, the intention is to bring the forehead to the knee rather than along the shin. To do this action the spine must flex very deeply, and there is less hip flexion than in the previous version. This action can be surprisingly difficult for people accustomed to forward bending from hip flexion rather than spinal flexion.

The shoulders are also more fully flexed, bringing them higher overhead, and adducted to bring the palms together. Rather than the palms resting on the floor, the fingertips reach out along the floor, sliding the little fingers away from the foot. Because the hands are not on the floor to either side of the foot, balancing in this pose is more challenging, though there is a clearer sense of midline with the hands pressing together.

Prasarita Padottanasana

Wide-Stance Forward Bend

pra-sa-REE-tah pah-doh-tahn-AHS-anna

prasarita = spread, expanded; *pada* = foot; *ut* = intense; *tan* = to stretch out

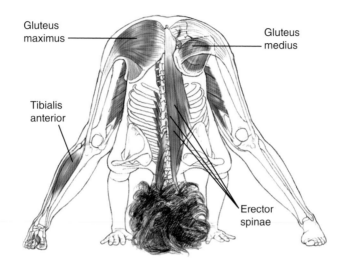

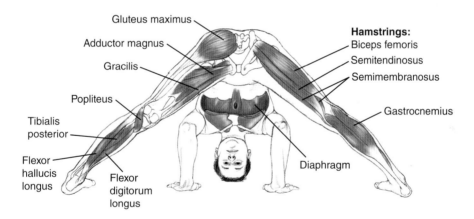

Classification

Symmetrical standing forward-bending pose

Skeletal joint actions	
Spine	**Lower limbs**
Mild flexion	Hip flexion and abduction, knee extension, ankle dorsiflexion, foot supination at heel and pronation at forefoot

(continued)

Muscular joint actions

Spine

Passively lengthening

Spinal muscles

Lower limbs

Concentric contraction	Eccentric contraction or passively lengthening
To extend knee: Articularis genu, vastii **To maintain arches of foot without inhibiting dorsiflexion of ankle:** Intrinsic muscles of foot	Hamstrings, especially medial hamstrings (semitendinosus and semimembranosus), adductor magnus and minimus, gracilis

Notes

This pose is often described as a stretch for the adductors or the muscles of the inner legs. In fact, when the legs are wide apart and the body is folded forward (hip adduction and flexion), some muscles of the adductor group are not lengthened at all, such as the pectineus and the anterior fibers of the adductor longus and brevis. This is because some adductors are also flexors and are not at their greatest length until the hip joints are adducted and extended, as when standing upright with the legs wide apart (if the pelvis isn't tipping forward, which would undo the hip extension and is a common pattern).

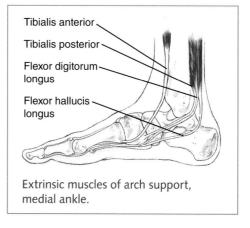

Extrinsic muscles of arch support, medial ankle.

Labels: Tibialis anterior, Tibialis posterior, Flexor digitorum longus, Flexor hallucis longus

When the stance is wide the feet need to be both strong and mobile in order to ground through the outer feet without overmobilizing the outer ankles or collapsing the inner ankles.

Breathing

Wide-stance forward bend is probably the safest, most accessible inversion in all of yoga practice. The more firmly the legs can create support while at the same time allowing the pelvis to freely rotate forward at the hip joints, the more relaxed the torso and breathing can be. This inversion provides mild traction and release to the spine while reversing the usual action of the breath.

Hanging upside down, the diaphragm is pulled cranially by gravity, thus favoring the exhalation and the venous return from the lower body. While inhaling, the diaphragm pushes the weight of the abdominal organs caudally (toward the tail) against gravity while at the same time mobilizing the costovertebral joints in the thoracic spine, which is being tractioned open. All these altered muscular actions can help normalize circulation in both muscles and organs that are constantly subjected to the usual stresses of upright weight bearing.

Upavesasana

Squat, Sitting-Down Pose

oo-pah-ve-SHAHS-anna

upavesa = sitting down, seat

This pose is almost never referred to by a Sanskrit name, but there is some precedent for the name given here.

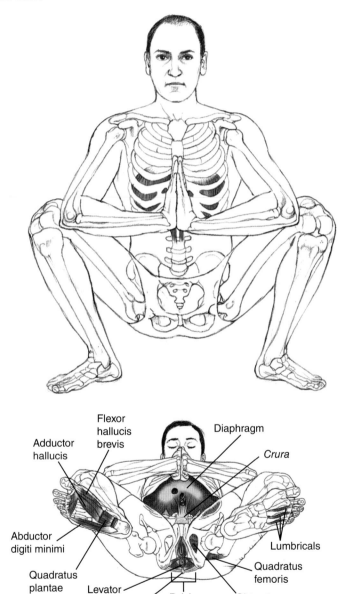

Adductor hallucis

Flexor hallucis brevis

Diaphragm

Crura

Abductor digiti minimi

Lumbricals

Quadratus plantae

Quadratus femoris

Levator ani

Coccyx

Pelvic floor

Obturator internus

Classification

Symmetrical standing pose

(continued)

Skeletal joint actions		
Spine	**Upper limbs**	**Lower limbs**
Axial extension	Slight shoulder flexion; elbow flexion; forearm pronation; wrist, hand, and finger extension	SI joint nutation; hip flexion, external rotation, and abduction; knee flexion; ankle dorsiflexion

Muscular joint actions	
Spine	
Concentric contraction	*Eccentric contraction*
To maintain arches of foot without inhibiting dorsiflexion of ankle:	**To allow hip flexion and support external rotation:**
Intrinsic muscles of foot	Gluteus maximus, piriformis, superior and inferior gemellus, obturator internus
	To allow hip and knee flexion and ankle dorsiflexion:
	Hamstrings at hip joint, vastii, soleus

Notes

For some people the pelvic floor can be contacted easily in this position, where it works synergistically to respond to the movement of the inhalation and to initiate the exhalation.

Gravity does the work of lowering the body down toward the floor, and the muscles of the legs are active to prevent collapsing completely into the joints. This is especially important in the hip joints, because if the weight of the upper body falls passively into the hip joints it may make the pelvic floor less accessible.

The inability to dorsiflex the ankles deeply enough to keep the heels on the floor can be due to shortness in the Achilles tendons (specifically the soleus in this position); however, restriction can also be in the front of the ankles. A quick fix is available by using support under the heels, but it's important not to become too reliant on it in case it prevents activation of the intrinsic muscles of the feet, which stabilize the arches, allow deeper flexion in the ankles, and align the bones of the feet and knee joints. Look for the tendons of the anterior tibialis popping forward; this is a sign that deep support is lacking. Let gravity create the flexion, and use the intrinsic muscles to maintain integrity.

Breathing

This pose offers an opportunity to powerfully lengthen all three curves of the spine (axial extension). By definition this usually engages all three bandhas, and in this position, the deep support in the arches of the feet energetically feeds into the lifting action of the pelvic floor and lower abdominal muscles (mula bandha). The bracing of the elbows against the knees allows for a strong lengthening of the thoracic spine and lifting of the base of the rib cage and respiratory diaphragm (uddiyana bandha). The action of jalandhara bandha, which flexes the head on the top of the spine to complete the action of axial extension, essentially freezes out the normal respiratory shape changes of breathing. This is when the unusual pattern of breath associated with mahamudra can arise deep in the core of the system (susumna).

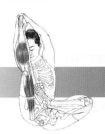

For many people in the industrialized world, sitting (or, more likely, slouching) on a piece of furniture is the body position in which they spend most of their waking hours. What shoes are to the feet, chairs, car seats, and couches are to the pelvic joints and lower spine.

In yoga practice, just as the bare feet develop a new relationship with the ground through the practice of standing asanas, the hips, pelvic joints, and lower spine develop a new relationship with the earth through bearing weight directly on them in sitting postures.

The asanas depicted in this chapter are either sitting positions themselves or are entered into from sitting. If practiced with attention to the anatomy of the relevant joints, muscles, and connective tissue, they can help to restore some of the natural flexibility that people had in childhood, when sitting and playing on the floor for hours at a time was effortless.

Beyond the idea of restoring natural function to the pelvis and lower back, yogic sitting also has an association with more advanced practices. The word *asana*, in fact, can be literally translated as "seat," and from a certain perspective, all of asana practice can be viewed as a methodical way of freeing up the spine, limbs, and breathing so that the yogi can spend extended periods of time in a seated position. In this most stable of upright body shapes, many of the distractions of dealing with gravity and balance can disappear, freeing the body's energies for the deeper contemplative work of meditative practices.

Note: Blue shaded areas indicate places of contact with the floor.

Sukhasana

Easy Posture

suk-HAS-anna

sukha = comfortable, gentle, agreeable

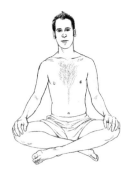 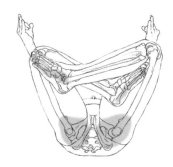

Siddhasana

Adept's Posture

sid-DHAS-anna

siddha = accomplished, fulfilled, perfected; a sage, an adept

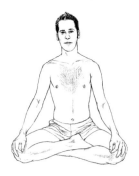 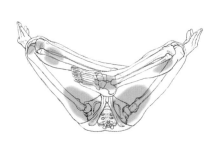

Svastikasana

Auspicious Posture

sva-steek-AHS-anna

svastik = lucky, auspicious

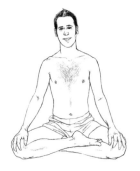 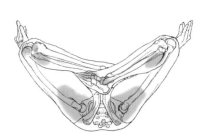

Padmasana

Lotus Posture

pod-MAHS-anna
padma = lotus

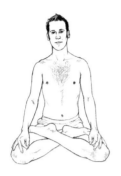
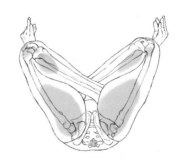

Mulabandhasana

Pose of the Root Lock

moola-ban-DHAS-anna
mula = root, foundation, bottom; *bandha* = binding, tying a bond

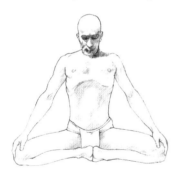
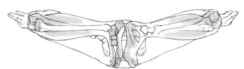

Common skeletal joint actions (for five previous poses)	
Spine	**Lower limbs**
Neutral or axial extension	Hip flexion, knee flexion

Notes

The goal of these seated poses is sthira and sukha—steadiness and ease. If the pelvis and legs are arranged in a way that clearly supports the spine, the spine can then be a support for the skull, and the spine and skull can together protect the brain and spinal cord. The nervous system can register this sense of support and ease, and turn its attention to practices such as pranayama or meditation.

When the spine is supported efficiently by the pelvis and legs, the ribs are also free to move with the breath, rather than become part of the supporting mechanism of sitting.

One thing to observe in the arrangements of the legs is to see if the knees are higher or lower than the hips. There are advantages and challenges in making either of these choices.

Sitting with the legs crossed in such a way that the knees are higher than the hip joints can be helpful for those who don't have a lot of external rotation or abduction in their hip joints (that is, if their knees don't fall open to the sides very easily). For these people, crossing the legs so the knees are higher than the hips can let the weight of the thigh bones settle deeply into the hip sockets and down into the ischial tuberosities (sitz bones).

If there is shortness in the back of the pelvis or hip joints, however, having the knees higher than the hips can tip the pelvis posteriorly and round the spine into flexion. To come to vertical it would then be necessary to engage the muscles of the spine or to contract the hip flexors to pull the pelvis and spine forward. This quickly becomes very tiring for the muscles of the back and of the front of the hip joints.

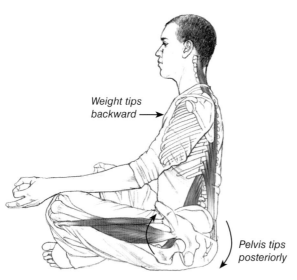

Weight tips backward

Pelvis tips posteriorly

Sitting with the knees above the hips can posteriorly rotate the pelvis and exaggerate primary curves.

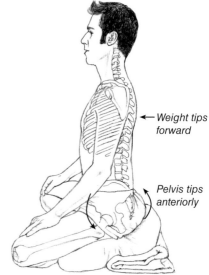

Weight tips forward

Pelvis tips anteriorly

Sitting with the hips above the knees can anteriorly tip the pelvis and exaggerate secondary curves.

128

Alternately, having the knees lower than the hips (by elevating the seat) prevents the pelvis from tipping backward and makes it easier to maintain the lumbar curve of the spine. The challenge in this arrangement of the legs is that it can tip someone too far forward on his sitz bones. The curves of the spine, particularly the lumbar curve, can be greatly exaggerated by this anterior tilt, and then the muscles of the back have to remain active to prevent falling forward.

In either case, tipping too far forward or too far backward necessitates using the muscles continuously to prevent falling into gravity.

The goal should be to find the position of the legs that allows the weight to fall most clearly from the spine through the pelvis into the sitz bones and the support of the floor, regardless of how high or low the knees are relative to the pelvis. In this way, a minimum amount of muscular effort is needed to align the bones for support. For some people this involves raising the seat a great deal or even sitting on a chair for ease in the spine until more mobility can be cultivated in the pelvis and legs. In a well-supported seated asana, the intrinsic equilibrium of the pelvis, spine, and breathing mechanism supports the body, and the energy that has been liberated from postural effort can be focused on deeper processes, such as breathing or meditation.

Dandasana

Staff Pose

dan-DAHS-anna

danda = stick, staff

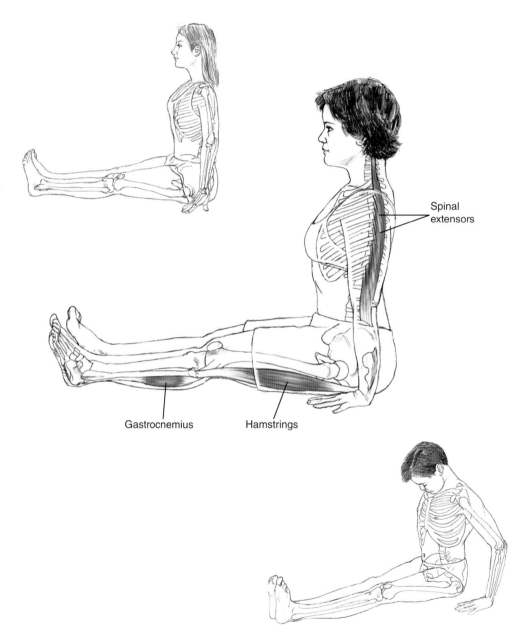

Spinal
extensors

Gastrocnemius   Hamstrings

Arm and torso proportions: short, neutral, and long.

Classification

Symmetrical seated pose

Skeletal joint actions		
Spine	**Upper limbs**	**Lower limbs**
Neutral or axial extension	Neutral scapula, shoulder adduction, elbow extension, wrist dorsiflexion	Hip flexion and adduction, knee extension, ankle dorsiflexion

Muscular joint actions

Spine

To calibrate concentric and eccentric contractions to maintain neutral alignment of spine:
Spinal extensors and flexors

Upper limbs

Concentric contraction

To resist adduction of scapula resulting from push of arm: Serratus anterior	**To extend elbow:** Triceps brachii

Lower limbs

Concentric contraction

To flex hip: Iliacus	**To extend knee:** Articularis genu, vastii
To adduct and internally rotate leg: Pectineus, adductor magnus	

Notes

While the legs are neutrally rotated in this position, against the pull of gravity most people need to actively use muscles of internal rotation to resist the legs falling open. This pose clearly reveals how tightness in the legs can create spinal flexion. Obstacles that show up in this pose are often the cause of difficulties in more complex poses, where the restrictions are less obvious. For example, tightness in the legs can affect downward-facing dog in a way that appears to be more about shoulder or spinal restriction.

Because proportional differences exist in arm-to-body length, not everyone can use the arms to help create the neutral spinal extension in dandasana. Conversely, what appear to be different arm-to-body proportions can sometimes be the result of chronically elevated or depressed positioning of the scapulae on the rib cage. In addition, if the spine is unable to extend into a vertical position because of tightness in the hips and legs, the arms may also seem too long.

Breathing

This is a straight-legged opportunity to breathe into an axially extended spine (mahamudra). All three bandhas can be employed here, and it is quite a challenge to take even 10 breaths while maintaining the bandhas with the spine in axial extension.

Paschimottanasana

West (Back) Stretching

POS-chee-moh-tan-AHS-anna

pascha = behind, after, later, westward; *uttana* = intense stretch

The back of the body is referred to as *west* because of the traditional practice of facing the rising sun when performing morning worship. Compare with purvottanasana, a stretch for the front of the body (*purva* = in front, before, eastward).

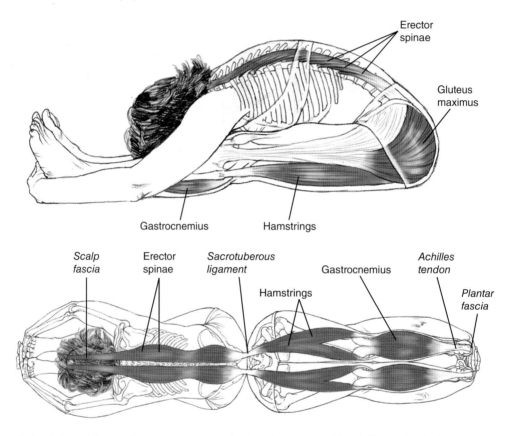

Erector spinae

Gluteus maximus

Gastrocnemius   Hamstrings

Scalp fascia   Erector spinae   Sacrotuberous ligament   Hamstrings   Gastrocnemius   Achilles tendon   Plantar fascia

The back line of the body is a continuous network of muscle and fascia that extends from the soles of the feet (plantar fascia) to the scalp fascia and the ridge of the brow.

Classification

Symmetrical seated forward-bending pose

Skeletal joint actions		
Spine	**Upper limbs**	**Lower limbs**
Mild flexion	Scapular abduction and upward rotation, shoulder flexion and adduction, elbow extension	SI joint nutation, hip flexion and adduction, knee extension, ankle dorsiflexion

Muscular joint actions	

Spine

Eccentric contraction

To distribute flexion through length of spine:
Spinal extensors

Upper limbs

Passively lengthening

Rhomboids, lower trapezius, latissimus dorsi

Lower limbs

Concentric contraction	*Passively lengthening*
To maintain knee extension: Articularis genu, vastii **To adduct and internally rotate:** Pectineus, adductor longus and brevis	Hamstrings, gluteus medius and minimus (posterior fibers), gluteus maximus, piriformis, adductor magnus, soleus, gastrocnemius

Notes

In this pose, gravity should do the work of moving you deeper into the forward bend; however, as the extensors of the spine lengthen, they are also actively distributing the action of flexion along the length of the spine, so that one part is not flexing excessively. If there is a lot of tightness in the back of the legs and pelvis, hip flexion is restricted and the hip flexors and abdominal muscles need to contract to pull the body forward, which can create a sense of congestion in the hip joints. Instead, elevate the seat with folded blankets or some other support under the sitz bones so that gravity can draw the upper body forward. Bending the knees can also allow the spine to come forward more easily. The hamstrings still lengthen, but in a less stressful way.

It should be noted that any stretching sensations close to the joints or at the points of attachment of a muscle indicate that the tendons and connective tissue are being stressed. Instead, the goal should be to direct the sensation along the whole length of a muscle rather than its attachment points.

The legs in this position are neither rotated internally nor externally. Many people, however, have a pattern of tightness in the back of the buttocks or legs that pulls the legs into external rotation. It is therefore important to engage the muscles of internal rotation to maintain neutral alignment.

Breathing

As in uttanasana (page 80), the standing version of this pose, deep hip flexion and spinal flexion compress the front of the body and restrict the ability of the abdomen to move with the breath. The more freedom in the rib cage, the easier it is to breathe in this position.

The breath can be very helpful while moving into this pose. The action of the exhalation can deepen flexion at the pelvis and hips when it is initiated with the lower abdominal muscles, and the action of the inhalation can assist in mobilizing the rib cage.

Janu Sirsasana

Head-to-Knee Pose

JAH-new shear-SHAHS-anna

janu = knee; *shiras* = to touch with the head

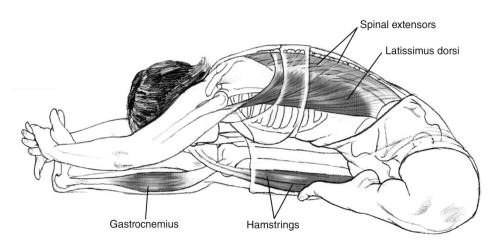

Spinal extensors

Latissimus dorsi

Gastrocnemius

Hamstrings

The entire back line of the extended leg side can be lengthened, from the sole of the foot to the scalp fascia.

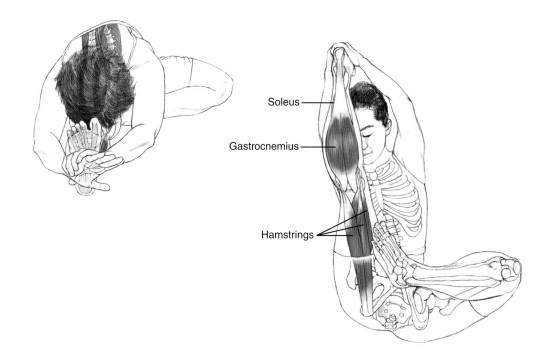

Soleus

Gastrocnemius

Hamstrings

Classification

Asymmetrical seated forward-bending pose

Skeletal joint actions

Spine	Upper limbs	Lower limbs	
		Extended leg	Flexed leg
Mild flexion, rotation of chest toward extended leg	Scapular abduction and upward rotation, shoulder flexion and adduction, elbow extension	SI joint nutation, hip flexion, knee extension, ankle dorsiflexion	SI joint nutation; hip flexion, external rotation, and abduction; knee flexion; ankle plantar flexion; foot supination

Muscular joint actions

Spine

Concentric contraction	Eccentric contraction
To rotate chest to face leg: Internal oblique (extended leg side); external oblique, rotatores, multifidi (flexed leg side)	**To facilitate rotation and distribute flexion through length of spine by lengthening eccentrically:** External oblique, rotatores, multifidi (extended leg side); internal oblique (flexed leg side)

Upper limbs

Concentric contraction	Passively lengthening
To upwardly rotate scapula: Serratus anterior **To flex and adduct arm:** Anterior deltoid, pectoralis major **To extend elbow:** Triceps brachii	Rhomboids, lower trapezius, latissimus dorsi

Lower limbs

Extended leg		Flexed leg	
Concentric contraction	Passively lengthening	Concentric contraction	Passively lengthening
To maintain knee extension: Articularis genu, vastii **To adduct and internally rotate:** Pectineus, adductor longus and brevis	Hamstrings, gluteus medius and minimus (posterior fibers), gluteus maximus, piriformis, adductor magnus, soleus, gastrocnemius	**To externally rotate and abduct hip:** Obturator internus and externus, quadratus femoris, piriformis, superior and inferior gemellus **To externally rotate and flex hip and knee:** Sartorius **To flex knee:** Hamstrings	Adductor magnus, longus, and brevis

(continued)

Notes

The asymmetry of this pose reveals how our preferences for habitually using one side of the body (our *sidedness*) is exhibited in the back muscles. Janu sirsasana can also reveal sidedness in the relative stability or mobility of the SI joints. Everyone has an "easy" and a "hard" side in this pose because of the inherent asymmetries of the human body.

The more mobile the SI joint is on the side of the flexed leg, the easier it is to turn and face the extended leg. This is especially true as the spine extends toward the extended leg. As hip flexion deepens, less spinal flexion is required. Because this further limits the rotation in the lumbar spine, more movement then needs to happen at the SI joint.

It is very common to overmobilize the SI joint in janu sirsasana. This happens when the pose is pushed or flexed too forcefully and movement is directed into one joint, rather than distributed through several joints. In this pose, as in many others, a little movement in a lot of places will give you the most range of motion without demanding too much movement in any single joint. To find this distribution of movement through the joints, it is important to identify the joints that move most easily (and encourage them to do less) and the joints that move less easily (and encourage them to do more).

Alternately, immobility of the pelvic joint can lead to excessive torque in the bent-leg knee joint. Many yogis report meniscus tears occurring as they move into this pose. This happens in a partially flexed knee as the pelvis flexes forward, taking the femur with it, which grinds the medial femoral condyle into the medial meniscus. Ensuring that the bent leg is truly fully flexed will move the meniscus safely to the back of the joint.

All this points to the fact that the potential stresses to the spine and SI, hip, and knee joints need to be evenly distributed so that no one structure takes all the force of this pose.

Breathing

The breath can be very helpful while moving into this pose. Emphasizing the action of the exhalation deepens the flexion at the pelvis, whereas emphasizing the action of the inhalation assists in extending the upper spine. This will only occur if the exhalation is initiated with the lower abdominal muscles and the inhalation is directed toward the rib cage.

It is interesting to experiment with the opposite pattern of breath just to create a contrast: Try exhaling by compressing the chest and inhaling into the belly region. Notice the effect on the asana compared with the first suggestions.

Parivrtta Janu Sirsasana

Revolved Head-to-Knee Pose

par-ee-vrt-tah JAH-new shear-SHAHS-anna

parivrtta = turning, rolling; *janu* = knee; *shiras* = to touch with the head

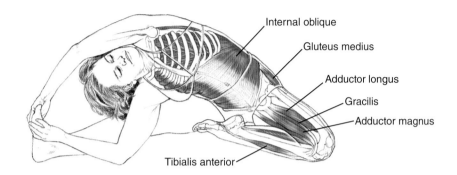

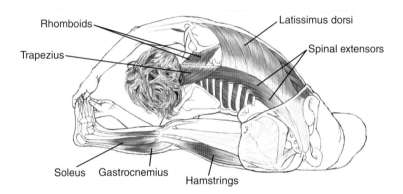

Classification

Asymmetrical seated side-bending pose

Skeletal joint actions			
Spine	**Upper limbs**	**Lower limbs**	
		Extended leg	**Flexed leg**
Lateral flexion, rotation away from extended leg	Scapular abduction, upward rotation, and elevation; shoulder abduction; elbow extension; forearm supination	Hip flexion, knee extension, ankle dorsiflexion	Hip flexion, external rotation, and abduction; knee flexion; ankle plantar flexion; foot supination

(continued)

Muscular joint actions

Spine

Concentric contraction	Eccentric contraction
To rotate chest to side:	**To modulate side bending into gravity:**
Internal oblique (flexed leg side); external oblique (extended leg side)	Quadratus lumborum, latissimus dorsi, spinal muscles (flexed leg side)
To rotate head toward ceiling:	
Rectus capitis posterior, obliquus capitis inferior, longus capitis and colli, splenius capitis (flexed leg side); sternocleidomastoid, upper trapezius (extended leg side)	

Upper limbs

Concentric contraction	Eccentric contraction
To upwardly rotate, abduct, and elevate scapula:	**To extend arm to overhead without falling into gravity:**
Serratus anterior	Rotator cuff, teres major, latissimus dorsi
To extend elbow:	
Triceps brachii, anconeus	

Lower limbs

Extended leg		Flexed leg	
Concentric contraction	Passively lengthening	Concentric contraction	Passively lengthening
To maintain knee extension:	Hamstrings, gluteus medius and minimus (posterior fibers), gluteus maximus, piriformis, adductor magnus, soleus, gastrocnemius	**To externally rotate hip:**	Adductor magnus, longus, and brevis
Articularis genu, vastii		Obturator internus and externus, quadratus femoris, piriformis, superior and inferior gemellus	
To adduct and internally rotate:		**To externally rotate and flex hip and knee:**	
Pectineus, adductor longus and brevis		Sartorius	
		To flex knee:	
		Hamstrings	

Notes

Although the legs in this pose are the same as in janu sirsasana (page 134), the action in the spine is very different: Instead of rotating toward the extended leg, the rotation is away from the leg, and instead of forward flexion in the spine, there is lateral flexion. This change in spinal action changes the action in the shoulder girdle and arms as well; notably, more lengthening occurs in the latissimus dorsi.

Side-bending poses are great for releasing restrictions in the shoulder joints. When flexion of the glenohumeral joint is restricted, greater mobility can often be found by mobilizing the scapula in lateral flexion.

In this pose, when the sitz bones stay on the floor the action of side bending is focused in the spine. If the sitz bone of the flexed leg is allowed to lift from the floor, the action of side bending moves further into the hip joint of the extended leg, and the back of that leg.

Breathing

The upper side of this pose is more expanded, and the rib cage is more open, but the lower dome of the diaphragm is more mobile, and the lower lung's tissue is more compliant. Focusing on this fact can quite naturally create a bit more awareness of the lower side, which helps prevent compressive collapse.

Mahamudra
The Great Seal
ma-ha-MOO-dra
maha = great, mighty, strong; *mudra* = sealing, shutting, closing

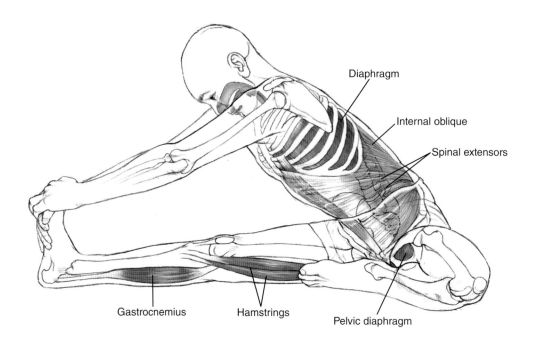

Diaphragm

Internal oblique

Spinal extensors

Gastrocnemius

Hamstrings

Pelvic diaphragm

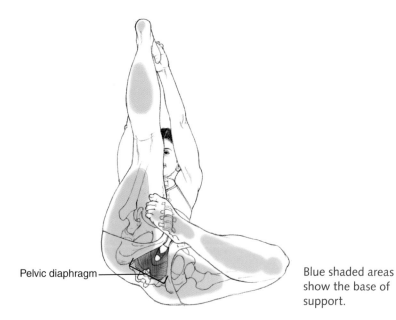

Pelvic diaphragm

Blue shaded areas show the base of support.

Classification

Asymmetrical seated axial extension pose

Skeletal joint actions

Spine	Upper limbs	Lower limbs	
		Extended leg	**Flexed leg**
Axial extension, rotation of chest toward extended leg	Scapular abduction and upward rotation, shoulder flexion and adduction, elbow extension	SI joint nutation, hip flexion, knee extension, ankle dorsiflexion	SI joint nutation; hip flexion, external rotation, and abduction; knee flexion; ankle plantar flexion; foot supination

Muscular joint actions

Spine

Concentric contraction	Eccentric contraction
To rotate chest to face leg and distribute axial extension: Internal oblique (extended leg side); external oblique, rotatores, multifidi (flexed leg side)	**To balance weight of head:** Posterior suboccipitals **To facilitate rotation and distribute axial extension through length of spine by lengthening eccentrically:** External oblique, rotatores, multifidi (extended leg side); internal oblique (flexed leg side)

Notes

The base of mahamudra is very similar to janu sirsasana (page 134), which it resembles, and the actions in the arms and legs are the same. However, the main action of the spine in this pose is strong axial spinal extension rather than spinal flexion.

A simplified way of thinking about this position is that it combines a forward bend (flexion of the lumbar and cervical spine), a backward bend (extension of the thoracic spine), and a twist (axial rotation of the thoracic spine and the turning of the pelvis toward the extended leg).

Breathing

Executing this pose properly while engaging all three bandhas is considered to be the ultimate test of the breath because mahamudra drives all the normal respiratory movements out of the body cavities: There is strong stabilizing action in the pelvic floor and abdominal muscles, the rib cage is held in a lifted position, the costovertebral joints are immobilized by thoracic twisting, and the sternum is lifted into the chin by the scalenes. All in all, the body is forced to find another, unusual way to breathe.

When all the usual, visible, external breath movements have been stabilized, something deep in the core of the system must mobilize through a new pathway. That pathway is commonly referred to in yogic literature as *susumna*—the central channel.

Upavistha Konasana

Seated Wide-Angle Pose

oo-pah-VEESH-tah cone-AHS-anna

upavistha = seated; *kona* = angle

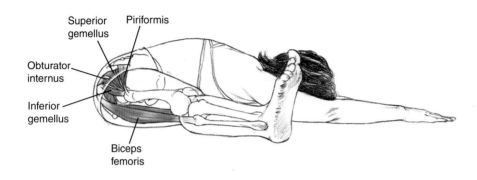

Superior gemellus

Piriformis

Obturator internus

Inferior gemellus

Biceps femoris

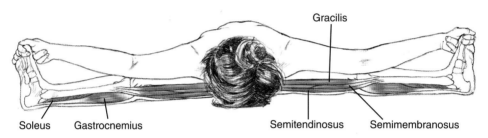

Gracilis

Soleus

Gastrocnemius

Semitendinosus

Semimembranosus

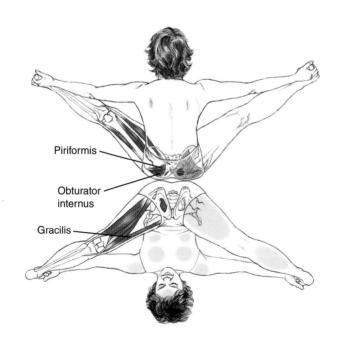

Piriformis

Obturator internus

Gracilis

Classification

Symmetrical seated forward-bending pose

Skeletal joint actions	
Spine	**Lower limbs**
Mild flexion moving toward axial extension	SI joint nutation, hip abduction and flexion, knee extension, ankle dorsiflexion

Muscular joint actions

Spine

Eccentric contraction
To distribute flexion through length of spine:
Spinal extensors

Lower limbs

Eccentric contraction	*Passively lengthening*
To abduct leg while folding forward in hip joint:	Gracilis
Gluteus medius and minimus, piriformis, superior and inferior gemellus, obturator internus	
To modulate forward bend:	
Semitendinosus, semimembranosus (medial hamstrings)	

Notes

Extensors of the spine are lengthening and active. As the pose deepens, the spine flattens to the floor and moves toward axial extension.

There is a strong action of nutation at the SI joints, as the top of the sacrum nods forward while leaving the iliac bones behind. If the sitz bones release from the floor, the action is more in the hip joints and back of the legs. If the sitz bones stay grounded, the action is distributed more evenly between the legs and spine.

The starting position of the legs is sometimes described as external rotation. If the feet point up to the ceiling, there is no external rotation in the hip joints. There is instead flexion and adduction at the hip joints.

If the legs roll inward, there can be too much lengthening for the inner knees and adductors. For tight students, it is preferable to bend the knees a bit (with support) so that the stretching sensations are felt more in the bellies of the relevant muscles. Sensations of stretch occurring near the joints and muscle attachments are indicators that nothing useful is likely to result from the movement.

Breathing

The act of gradually lengthening the spine in this pose can be greatly assisted by the breath. The exhalation, if initiated in the lower abdomen, can help anchor the sitting bones and ground the backs of the thighs, whereas the inhalation, if it's initiated in the upper chest, can help to lengthen the spine. In short, the exhalation can ground the posture's lower half, and the inhalation can lengthen the posture's upper half.

Baddha Konasana

Bound Angle Pose

BAH-dah cone-AHS-anna

baddha = bound; *kona* = angle

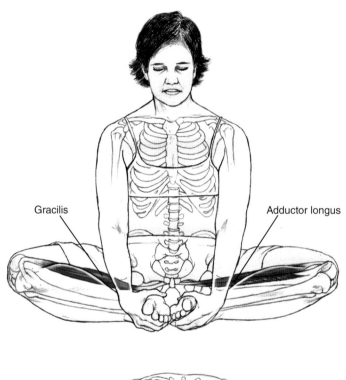

Gracilis

Adductor longus

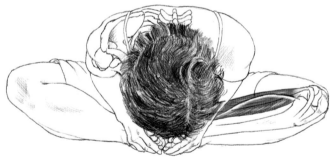

Classification

Symmetrical seated forward-bending pose

Skeletal joint actions	
Spine	**Lower limbs**
Mild flexion moving toward axial extension	SI joint nutation; hip flexion, external rotation, and adduction; knee flexion; ankle dorsiflexion; foot supination

Muscular joint actions

Spine

Eccentric contraction

To distribute flexion through length of spine:
Spinal extensors

Lower limbs

Eccentric contraction	*Passively lengthening*
To externally rotate hip:	Adductor magnus, longus, and brevis; gracilis
Obturator internus and externus, quadratus femoris, piriformis, superior and inferior gemellus	

Notes

Much as in paschimottanasana (page 132), if the focus is too much on getting the head down, the resulting action is more spinal (flexion) than pelvic (SI and hip joints). For this reason, the intention should not be to get the head to the feet, but to get the navel to the feet.

The activity of the obturator internus in this pose also activates the muscles of the pelvic floor, which can anchor the base of the pose.

Depending on how close the feet are to the groin, different external rotators are activated to assist with rotating the legs out, and different adductors are lengthened. The more the knees are extended, the more the gracilis is lengthened. Because the adductor longus and brevis work to flex and externally rotate the leg, the abduction in the pose lengthens these two muscles of the adductor group. Thus, it's quite valuable to work with the feet at different distances from the pelvis. Closer isn't always better.

Baddha konasana can be challenging for the knees. The supination of the feet (soles toward the ceiling) causes a rotation of the tibia that, combined with flexion, destabilizes the ligamentous support for the knees. If the hips are not very mobile and the legs are pushed into this pose, the lower leg torque can travel into the knee joints. One way to protect them is to evert the feet (press the outer edges into the floor). This activates the peroneal muscles, which, via fascial connections, can stabilize the lateral ligaments of the knees and help to keep them from rotating too much. The result is that more of the pose's action is directed into the hip joints.

Breathing

The advice to bring the navel—rather than the head—to the feet is another way of minimizing obstructions to the breath. Pushing the head toward the floor collapses the rib cage and compresses the abdomen, resulting in a reduced ability for those cavities to change shape. A lengthened spine results in freer breathing.

(continued)

Baddha Konasana Variation

Supta Baddha Konasana
Reclining Bound Angle Pose

supta = resting, lain down to sleep; *baddha* = bound; *kona* = angle

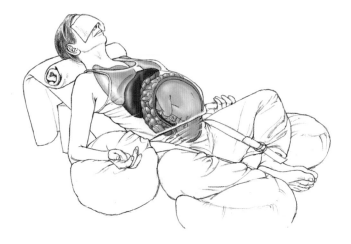

Notes

This restful variation of baddha konasana puts the spine in neutral alignment or very mild extension to gently open up the breathing. It is a very commonly used restorative posture. With the use of props such as bolsters, blankets, straps, and cushions, it can be modified in a wide variety of ways.

Kurmasana

Turtle Pose

koor-MAHS-anna

kurma = tortoise, turtle

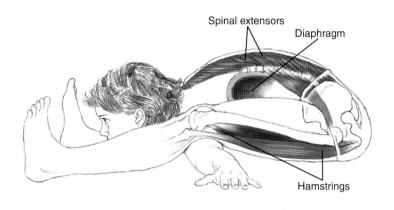

Spinal extensors

Diaphragm

Hamstrings

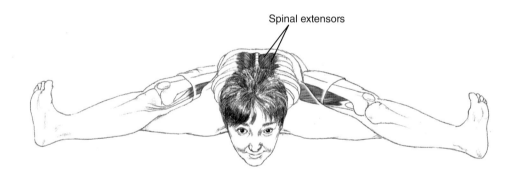

Spinal extensors

Classification

Symmetrical seated forward-bending pose

Skeletal joint actions		
Spine	**Upper limbs**	**Lower limbs**
Cervical extension, thoracic and lumbar flexion moving toward extension	Scapular downward rotation and abduction, shoulder abduction and internal rotation, elbow extension, forearm pronation	SI joint nutation, hip flexion and abduction, knee extension, ankle dorsiflexion

(continued)

Muscular joint actions	

Spine

Concentric contraction	*Eccentric contraction*
To extend spine against resistance of position of leg and arm: Spinal extensors	**To resist hyperextending cervical spine:** Neck flexors

Upper limbs

Concentric contraction	*Eccentric contraction*
To internally rotate and protect shoulder joint: Rotator cuff (especially subscapularis) **To adduct scapula once arm is under leg:** Rhomboids, trapezius **To press arm against leg:** Posterior deltoid	**To resist hyperextension in elbow:** Biceps brachii

Lower limbs

Concentric contraction	*Eccentric contraction*
To extend knee over arm: Articularis genu, vastii **To adduct and internally rotate leg:** Pectineus, adductor longus and brevis	**To press leg into arm while modulating forward bend:** Gluteus medius and minimus, piriformis, superior and inferior gemellus, obturator internus, hamstrings

Notes

To prepare for this pose, the spine flexes, the scapulae abduct, the hips flex and abduct, and the knees flex. Once the arms are in position under the legs, the actions that deepen the pose are the reversal of the preparatory ones: spinal extension, scapular adduction, hip extension and adduction, and knee extension.

This opposition of actions in the spine and scapulae means that muscles such as the spinal extensors and rhomboids are asked to contract from a very lengthened position (one of the more challenging positions from which to concentrically contract a muscle).

Because the arms are bound under the legs, the action can potentially be forced into vulnerable spots: The spine could overflex in the lumbar or thoracic regions, or the hamstrings could overmobilize at their attachment on the sitz bones.

Breathing

The diaphragm receives considerable compression when entering into this position, and the gradual movement out of thoracic flexion can be seen as an attempt to reestablish the breathing space in the thoracic cavity.

Kurmasana Variation

Supta Kurmasana

Reclining Turtle Pose

supta = reclining; *kurma* = tortoise, turtle

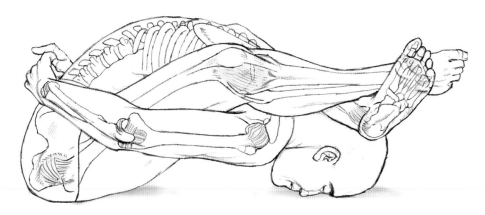

Joint capsules are shaded in blue.

Notes

This pose can be very intense or of great ease. With the arms and legs bound, little work is needed to maintain the position if enough range of motion exists in all the joints of the body to enter the pose. If the action is not distributed through all the joints, this pose has the potential for directing too much force into the spine, the SI joints, and, with the arms bound in this position, the fronts of the shoulder joints. The rotator cuff (especially the subscapularis) is working to both internally rotate the humerus and protect the joint from protraction.

The more freedom there is in the scapulae gliding on the rib cage, the less force is directed into the glenohumeral joints and their capsules. Using the latissimus dorsi to help internally rotate and extend the arms interferes with the flexion of the spine, because the latissimus dorsi are also spinal extensors.

The bound position of the legs behind the skull and cervical spine creates potential stress in this area, too, either overstretching the back of the neck or overworking the muscles against the push of the legs.

If there isn't enough mobility in the rest of the spine, the cervical spine can be overflexed to get the legs in position. This should be avoided.

Breathing

Once locked into this bound pose, the abdominal muscles don't have much to do, so they can be released for belly breaths. This is actually advisable, because excessive thoracic action during trunk flexion can stress an already vulnerable neck.

Ardha Matsyendrasana

Half Lord of the Fishes Pose

ARD-hah MOTS-yen-DRAHS-anna

ardha = half; *matsya* = fish; *indra* = ruler, lord
Sage Matsyenda was a renowned teacher of yoga who, according to legend, developed this pose.

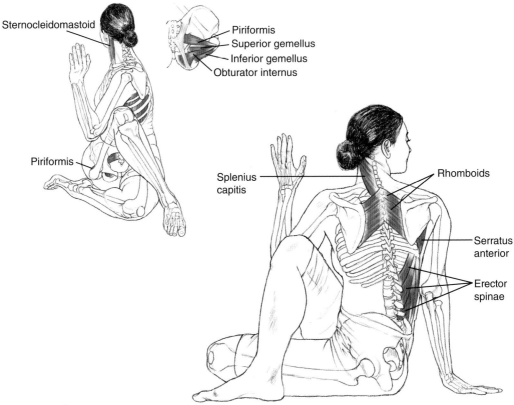

Classification

Asymmetrical seated twisting pose

Skeletal joint actions				
Spine	**Upper limbs**		**Lower limbs**	
	Front arm (contralateral to top leg)	**Back arm**	**Top leg**	**Bottom leg**
Rotation toward top leg	Neutral scapula, shoulder abduction, elbow flexion	Shoulder extension, elbow extension, wrist dorsiflexion	Hip flexion and adduction, knee flexion, foot on floor	Hip flexion, external rotation, and adduction; knee flexion; ankle plantar flexion

Muscular joint actions

Spine

Concentric contraction	Passively lengthening
To maintain extension against pressure of arm: Spinal extensors **To rotate spine toward leg:** Internal oblique, erector spinae, splenius capitis (top leg side); external oblique, rotatores, multifidi (bottom leg side) **To turn head:** Sternocleidomastoid (bottom leg side)	External oblique, rotatores, multifidi, sternocleidomastoid (top leg side); internal oblique, erector spinae, splenius capitis, latissimus dorsi (bottom leg side)

Upper limbs

Front arm (contralateral to top leg)	Back arm
Concentric contraction	*Concentric contraction*
To stabilize humeral head: Rotator cuff **To maintain placement of scapula on rib cage:** Rhomboids **To extend arm against leg:** Posterior deltoid **To flex elbow:** Biceps brachii	**To stabilize humeral head:** Rotator cuff **To keep scapula placed on rib cage and resist adduction of this scapula:** Serratus anterior **To extend shoulder and elbow:** Triceps brachii

Lower limbs

Top leg		Bottom leg	
Concentric contraction	*Passively lengthening*	*Concentric contraction*	*Passively lengthening*
To flex and adduct leg: Adductor longus and brevis, pectineus	Piriformis; superior and inferior gemellus; obturator internus and externus; quadratus femoris; gluteus maximus, medius, and minimus	**To externally rotate hip:** Obturator internus and externus, quadratus femoris, piriformis, superior and inferior gemellus **To externally rotate and flex hip and knee:** Sartorius **To flex knee:** Hamstrings **To flex and adduct leg:** Adductor longus and brevis	Gluteus medius and minimus

(continued)

Notes

All parts of the torso can contribute to this twist—both right and left sides of the front and both right and left sides of the back, at different layers of muscle. The spine has the most balanced rotation when in neutral extension. Flexion in the lumbar spine jeopardizes the stability of the lumbar vertebrae and discs, and too much extension tends to lock the thoracic spine into place, inhibiting axial rotation there.

You can fake the twisting action of this pose by overmobilizing the scapulae and allowing them to adduct (the back one) and abduct (the front one) excessively. When this happens you see the appearance of rotation, but not much actual movement in the spine. Because the shoulder girdle has more range of motion in this direction than the thoracic structures have, it is frequently a more intense spinal twist when the arms are placed in a simple, non-bound position. If you would like to clarify the action of the spine, enter this pose without using the arms so the maximum safe action is found in the spine. The leverage of the arms can come in last as a deepening action. Overuse of the arms can direct too much force into vulnerable parts of the spine, particularly T11 and T12.

Another factor that contributes to the intensity of the spinal twisting action of this pose is the arrangement of the legs, which greatly limits rotational movements in the pelvis—and in fact counterrotates the pelvis away from the rotation of the spine.

Breathing

Ardha matsyendrasana provides a very clear opportunity to explore the basic dynamics of the breath as they relate to the principles of brhmana and langhana, prana and apana, and sthira and sukha.

The lower body is the stable base of the pose, and a langhana (belly breathing) pattern can release tension in the lower abdomen, hip joints, and pelvic floor. This approach to breathing stimulates the experience of apana flowing downward in the system, into the earth.

The upper body is the mobile, supported aspect of the pose, and the brhmana (chest breath) can be accomplished here simply by stabilizing the abdominal wall upon the initiation of the inhalation. This moves the diaphragm's action into the rib cage and costovertebral articulations and greatly intensifies deep rotational release in the thoracic spine. This breathing pattern is clearly related to the upward movement of apana, using the lower abdominal muscles to assist in driving the exhalation upward and outward from the body.

In this pose, use a simple nonbound arm position and try doing several rounds of relaxed belly breathing to begin with. Then, gradually deepen the lower abdominal contractions on the exhalation, eventually maintaining each contraction for a moment when initiating the next inhalation. Notice the effect of the breathing patterns on your experience of the pose.

Gomukhasana

Cow-Faced Pose

go-moo-KAHS-anna

go = cow; *mukha* = face

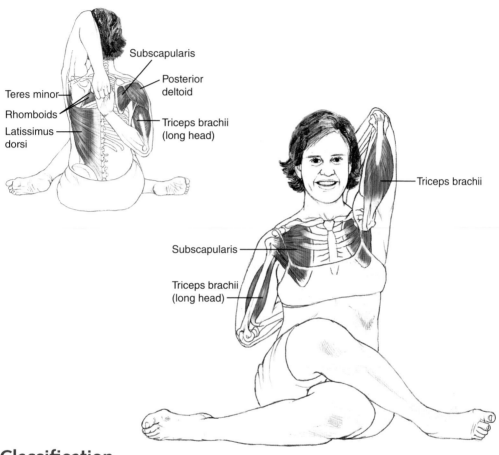

Classification

Asymmetrical seated pose

Skeletal joint actions			
Spine	**Upper limbs**		**Lower limbs**
	Top arm	**Bottom arm**	
Neutral spine with slight extension in thoracic spine	Scapular upward rotation, elevation, and adduction; shoulder external rotation and flexion; elbow flexion; forearm pronation	Scapular downward rotation, adduction, and depression; shoulder internal rotation and extension; elbow flexion; forearm supination	Hip flexion, external rotation, and adduction; knee flexion

(continued)

Muscular joint actions

Spine

To calibrate concentric and eccentric contractions and to maintain neutral alignment of spine:
Spinal extensors and flexors

Upper limbs

Top arm		Bottom arm	
Concentric contraction	*Passively lengthening*	*Concentric contraction*	*Passively lengthening*
To upwardly rotate scapula: Serratus anterior **To adduct scapula:** Rhomboids **To externally rotate shoulder:** Infraspinatus, teres minor **To flex arm overhead:** Anterior deltoid **To pronate forearm:** Pronator teres	Triceps brachii, latissimus dorsi, teres major, pectoralis minor	**To downwardly rotate and adduct scapula:** Lower trapezius, rhomboids **To internally rotate shoulder:** Subscapularis **To internally rotate and extend shoulder:** Teres major, latissimus dorsi **To extend arm:** Triceps brachii (long head), posterior deltoid **To flex elbow:** Biceps brachii **To supinate forearm:** Supinators	Biceps brachii (long head), pectoralis major, serratus anterior, upper trapezius

Lower limbs

Concentric contraction	*Passively lengthening*
To externally rotate hip: Obturator internus and externus, quadratus femoris, piriformis, superior and inferior gemellus **To externally rotate and flex hip and knee:** Sartorius **To flex knee:** Hamstrings **To flex and adduct leg:** Adductor longus and brevis	Gluteus medius and minimus

Notes

Upward and downward rotation of the scapula needs to precede adduction to avoid over-mobilizing the shoulder joint. If the scapula doesn't mobilize, there can be too much movement in the glenohumeral joint, causing overmobilizing in the joint capsule or impingements in the tendons of the biceps brachii and supraspinatus.

If the hip joints are not sufficiently mobile, excessive torque can result in the knee joints. Great care should be taken to avoid any strain in the knees, because the menisci are most vulnerable when the knee joints are semiflexed.

Breathing

Releasing the abdominal wall and directing the breath into the lower abdomen help the pelvic floor and hip joints to release. Restraining the lower abdomen during an inhalation directs the breath into the thoracic region, which intensifies the movement in the shoulder structures.

Hanumanasana

Monkey Pose

ha-new-mahn-AHS-anna

hanumat = having large jaws; a monkey chief

Hanuman was the semidivine chief of an army of monkeys who served the god Rama. As told in the Hindu epic *Ramayana* through the oral tradition, Hanuman once jumped in a single stride the distance between Southern India and (Sri) Lanka. This split-leg pose mimics his famous leap.

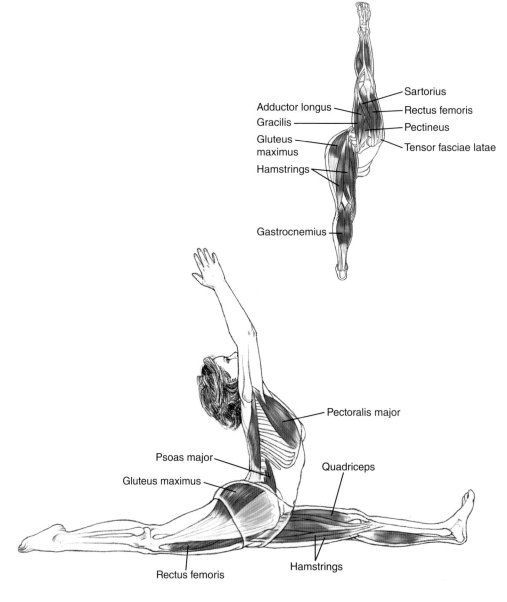

Classification

Asymmetrical seated forward-bending and backward-bending pose

Skeletal joint actions

Spine	Upper limbs	Lower limbs	
		Front leg	Back leg
Extension	Scapular upward rotation, abduction, and elevation; shoulder flexion and adduction; elbow extension	SI joint nutation; hip flexion, internal rotation, and adduction; knee extension; ankle dorsiflexion	SI joint counternutation; hip extension, internal rotation, and adduction; knee extension; ankle plantar flexion

Muscular joint actions

Spine

Concentric contraction	Eccentric contraction
To extend spine: Spinal extensors	**To allow spinal extension (back bending) without falling into gravity:** Psoas minor, abdominal muscles, longus colli, verticalis, suprahyoid and infrahyoid muscles

Upper limbs

Concentric contraction	Passively lengthening
To abduct, upwardly rotate, and elevate scapula: Serratus anterior, upper trapezius **To stabilize, flex, and adduct shoulder joint:** Rotator cuff, coracobrachialis, pectoralis major (upper fibers), anterior deltoid, biceps brachii (short head)	Rhomboids, latissimus dorsi, pectoralis major (lower fibers), pectoralis minor

Lower limbs

Front leg		Back leg
Concentric contraction	Eccentric contraction	Eccentric contraction
To maintain knee extension: Articularis genu, vastii **To adduct and internally rotate:** Pectineus, adductor longus and brevis	**To resist overarticulating in front hip joint and to maintain internal rotation and adduction:** Hamstrings, gluteus medius and minimus (posterior fibers), gluteus maximus, piriformis, adductor magnus, soleus, gastrocnemius	**To resist overextension of hip while maintaining adduction and internal rotation:** Psoas major, iliacus, rectus femoris, sartorius, pectineus, adductor longus and brevis, gracilis, tensor fasciae latae

(continued)

Notes

In this extreme pose, the forward-bending action in the front leg and pelvic half is countered by the backward-bending action in the back leg and pelvic half. The spine can then seek balance between those two opposing actions.

In a symmetrical forward bend like paschimottanasana (page 132), part of the action of forward bending comes from the spine, as well as the lower limbs. Similarly, in a back bend like urdhva dhanurasana (page 249), the backward-bending action comes from the lower limbs and spine together. In hanumanasana, however, the fact that the two legs are doing opposite actions means that the forward-bending and backward-bending actions are directed almost totally into the legs, making both aspects more intense.

Because there is generally more range of motion for the hip joint in flexion than in extension, the front leg usually moves more quickly into flexion and the movement of the back leg draws the spine into extension. This is also why more work is often felt in the extensors of the front leg than in the flexors of the back leg. The action in each leg is limited by the opposite leg, making it a kind of bound pose. This limitation means that force isn't dispersed into space so much as directed into potentially vulnerable areas (hamstring attachments are especially at risk for overmobilizing in this pose). This concern is greatly compounded if the pose is done passively.

The presence of gravity means that it isn't necessary to concentrically contract any muscles to pull the body into this position; instead, the weight of the body itself deepens the action. To do the pose safely, however, the body is not just passively releasing into gravity.

If hanumanasana is done more actively, with attention to the eccentric actions of the lengthening muscles, the mobilization of the pose can be distributed over several joints; a little movement in a lot of places can safely distribute the force. This requires awareness of your own tendencies toward places you hold or let go so that you can stabilize the mobile spots and mobilize the fixated areas.

A final note about having the legs in neutral rotation: While the position of the legs is neutral in terms of internal and external rotation, it actually takes active internal rotation to maintain this neutral position. A neutral position in the joint is not always the position with the least muscular effort, depending on the actions of gravity and the other limbs. Maintaining a neutral position can often be a quite vigorous action muscularly.

In this pose, many people let the back leg externally rotate to get it all the way down. Letting the back leg roll out puts twisting pressure into the lumbar spine and the SI joint of the back leg, not to mention a twisting pressure into the back knee. It also puts more pressure into the adductors of the back leg (adductor longus and brevis, pectineus, and gracilis) without the eccentric support of the iliacus and psoas major or rectus femoris. As a result, the groin can be overmobilized, and the usually overtight rectus femoris doesn't get as much movement as it could. It takes a different kind of discipline to resist the impulse to go as low as possible and to use props (blocks and blankets) as necessary to maintain the integrity of the pose.

Breathing

You'll know you're doing this pose effectively when you can breathe freely. Until all the flexion, extension, and rotational forces have been neutralized and the spine can extend easily, the breathing tends to be labored and rough. The use of props is highly recommended so that the work can be done in a gradual way that doesn't excessively disturb the rhythm of the breath.

Navasana

Boat Pose

nah-VAHS-anna

nava = boat

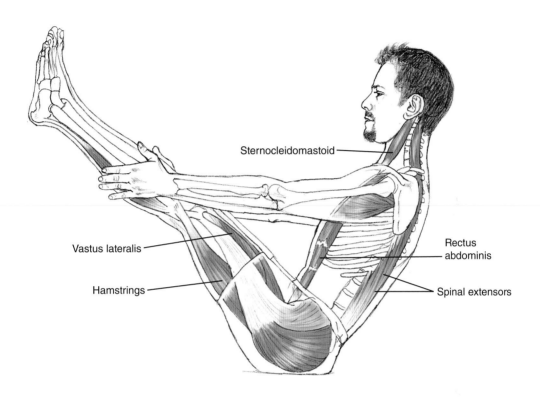

Sternocleidomastoid

Vastus lateralis

Hamstrings

Rectus abdominis

Spinal extensors

Classification

Symmetrical forward-bending balancing pose

Skeletal joint actions		
Spine	**Upper limbs**	**Lower limbs**
Neutral spine	Shoulder flexion	Hip flexion and adduction, knee extension

(continued)

Muscular joint actions	

Spine

Concentric contraction	*Eccentric contraction*
To maintain neutral curves of spine: Spinal extensors	**To maintain neutral spine against pull of gravity and resist hyperextension of lumbar spine:** Psoas major (upper fibers), abdominal muscles

Upper limbs

Concentric contraction	
To hold scapula on rib cage: Serratus anterior, rhomboids **To flex shoulder:** Coracobrachialis, anterior deltoid	**To extend elbow:** Triceps brachii, anconeus

Lower limbs

Concentric contraction	
To flex hip: Psoas major, iliacus, rectus femoris **To maintain knee extension:** Articularis genu, vastii	**To adduct and internally rotate:** Pectineus, gracilis, adductor longus and brevis

Notes

In this pose the challenge is not the position itself so much as its relationship to gravity. If it were rotated 45 degrees, it would be the work of sitting vertically in dandasana (which can certainly present its own challenges; see page 130).

Ideally, the weight in this pose is distributed between the sitting bones and the tailbone. All the weight should not be borne on the sacrum. If dandasana is a challenge because of shortness in the backs of the legs, that same shortness makes it impossible to support navasana correctly with the legs straight. In this case, bending the knees so that the spine can remain neutral is a good option.

This asana is often said to work the abdominal muscles. This is true; however, the abdominal muscles do not pull the body into this pose—rather, they are keeping the upper body from falling back into gravity. The action that holds the body in this position is hip flexion, created by the psoas major and iliacus. If the psoas major and iliacus are difficult to access, it is possible to overwork the rectus femoris or tensor fasciae latae attempting to stay up.

Just as bending the knees makes this pose easier by shortening the length of the lower lever arm, extending the arms overhead makes it more difficult by lengthening the upper lever arm.

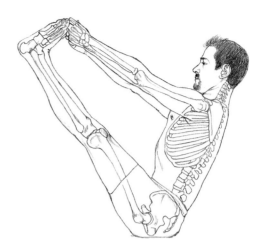

Navasana with arms extended.

Breathing

To maintain the stability and balance of this pose, the breath must be very restrained and focused. To illustrate how vital this is, attempt to do navasana while taking deep belly breaths.

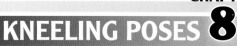
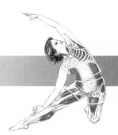

KNEELING POSES 8

When kneeling, the body's weight is on the knees, shins, and tops of the feet. Kneeling brings the center of gravity closer to the ground than standing, but farther from the ground than sitting. Kneeling, which includes both kneel-sitting and kneel-standing, is an important transitional place for babies learning to move from sitting to standing.

This position is associated with lowering oneself in the sense of meekness or worship. This probably evolved from the fact that when kneeling, a person is more vulnerable than when standing, especially if their head is bowed. Even the proud, upright stance of kings and pharaohs is tempered by their depiction in this humble position when they are at worship.

Kneeling is also a posture of relaxed alertness that is associated with strength and readiness, as seen in vajrasana and virasana (page 164). In martial arts, kneeling is used as a preparatory position that is easier to stand from more quickly than sitting cross-legged, and in the practice of aikido they even train to do throws from kneeling.

In asana, kneeling poses are often used to help mobilize the hip joints. When the mobility of the feet and lower legs is removed from the base of support, attention can be focused on the actions in the hip joints, pelvic halves, and pelvic floor.

Kneeling also provides a stable and symmetrical base from which the center of gravity can be raised up so the spine can fully extend, most beautifully expressed in poses such as ustrasana (page 170) and eka pada rajakapotasana (page 172).

Vajrasana

Thunderbolt Posture

vahj-RAHS-anna

vajra = thunderbolt, diamond

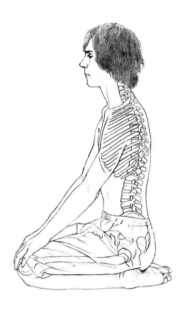
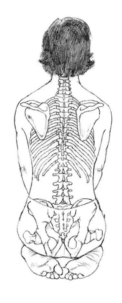
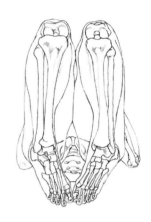

Virasana

Hero's Posture

veer-AHS-anna

vira = man, hero, chief

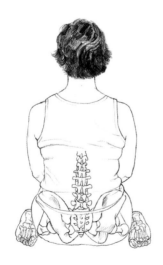
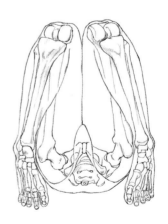

Common skeletal joint actions (for two previous poses)	
Spine	**Lower limbs**
Neutral or axial extension	Hip flexion, internal rotation, and adduction; knee flexion; ankle plantar flexion

Notes

As in sitting poses such as sukhasana (page 126), siddhasana (page 126), and padmasana (page 127), the goal is steadiness and ease, or sthira and sukha, the fundamental qualities of all asanas as described by Patañjali in the *Yoga Sutras*. Virasasana and vajrasana are excellent poses for supporting the spine and skull in a way that allows the senses to turn inward for pranayama and meditation (like the sitting poses beginning on page 126).

For some people, these kneeling positions are easier than sitting cross-legged because the hip joints do not need to externally rotate or adduct as they do in siddhasana or sukhasana.

Kneeling poses are also more symmetrical because both legs can do the same action and neither leg is crossed in front of the other. This crossing of the legs creates an asymmetrical action in the pelvis and hips that can have long-term effects.

Balasana

Child's Pose

bah-LAHS-anna

bala = young, childish, not fully grown or developed

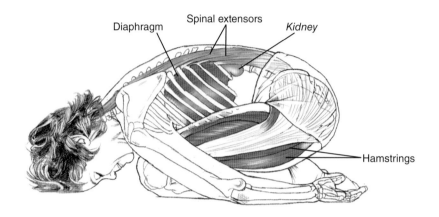

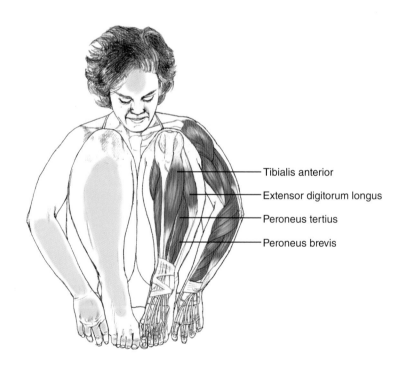

Classification

Symmetrical kneeling forward-bending pose

Skeletal joint actions	
Spine	**Lower limbs**
Flexion	SI joint nutation, hip flexion and adduction, knee flexion, ankle plantar flexion

Notes

Gravity draws the yielding body deeper into this position.

One goal of this pose is to bring the sitting bones to the heels and the forehead to the floor. To do so, many muscles have to lengthen: the extensors of the spine, gluteus maximus, piriformis and other rotators, hamstrings, gluteus medius and minimus (because of hip adduction), tibialis anterior, peroneus tertius, extensor digitorum longus and brevis, and extensor hallucis longus and brevis in the feet.

Variations include widening the knees (hip abduction), which can create more neutral extension in the spine and make room for the belly; extending the arms overhead; clasping the heels with the hands; crossing the arms under the forehead; and turning the head to one side.

Sometimes there is congestion in the fronts of the hip joints. It can be caused by using the hip flexors to pull the body down toward the thighs, rather than allowing gravity to create that action. The use of props can assist in this release.

If the extensors of the toes are tight or if there is a lack of mobility in the bones of the feet, restriction can also be felt in the tops of the feet. In addition, weakness in the intrinsic muscles of the feet often results in cramping in this and similar positions (such as virasana and vajrasana, page 164).

Breathing

With the hips fully flexed and adducted and the front of the torso resting on the anterior surfaces of the thighs, the movement of the breath in the abdomen and anterior rib cage is greatly restricted. This necessitates more movement in the back of the waist and rib cage. That is why if tightness exists in those places, this pose can feel suffocating.

Supta Virasana
Reclining Hero Pose
soup-tah veer-AHS-anna

supta = reclining, lain down to sleep; *vira* = a brave or eminent man, hero, chief

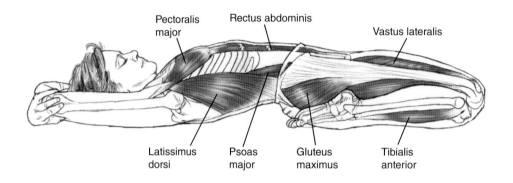

Pectoralis major · Rectus abdominis · Vastus lateralis · Latissimus dorsi · Psoas major · Gluteus maximus · Tibialis anterior

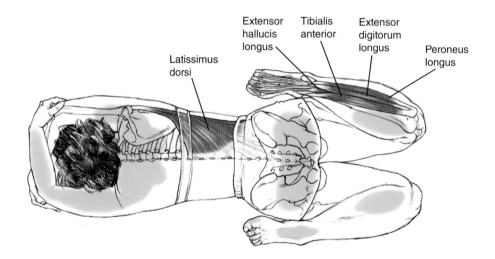

Extensor hallucis longus · Tibialis anterior · Extensor digitorum longus · Peroneus longus · Latissimus dorsi

Classification
Symmetrical kneeling backward-bending pose

Skeletal joint actions	
Spine	**Lower limbs**
Axial extension	SI joint counternutation; hip extension, internal rotation, and adduction; knee flexion and medial rotation; ankle plantar flexion

Muscular joint actions	

Spine

Concentric contraction	Passively lengthening
To prevent overmobilization of lumbar spine: Psoas minor, abdominal muscles	Psoas major

Lower limbs

Concentric contraction	Passively lengthening
To keep knees together: Gracilis, adductor magnus	Psoas major, rectus femoris, vastii, sartorius, tibialis anterior, extensor digitorum longus, extensor hallucis longus

Notes

Many variations exist for the arm position in this pose—at the sides, reaching overhead, and propped up on the elbows. If the latissimus dorsi are short, reaching the arms overhead can cause hyperextension of the spine because of the attachment of the latissimus dorsi in the lower back.

Because hip extension in internal rotation is generally more challenging than in external rotation, supta virasana reveals how open the "groins" truly are. This pose often begins as spinal extension, especially if there is tightness in the hip flexors, because the internal rotation of the legs is bound into place by the weight of the body.

If the hip extensors are tight and the pose is forced, the force can be transmitted either into the lower back or into the knees. The pose should instead be supported in a way that allows for maximum hip extension; getting down to the floor is less important.

Because the knees are at risk, keeping the feet active and avoiding supination is important for maintaining integrity in the knee joints.

This can be an excellent pose for sciatic and low-back pain if done with attention to the internal rotation and extension in the hips. If poorly executed, the pose can exacerbate low-back pain.

Breathing

The tautness in the psoas major and abdominal wall creates both posterior and anterior pressure in the abdominal cavity. This effect is magnified when activating the abdominal muscles to flatten the lumbar curve. The resulting breathing patterns would favor movements above and below the abdominal pressure.

Emphasizing thoracic breath movements at the base of the rib cage helps to mobilize the upper spine and shoulder girdle. Focusing on pelvic floor movements assists in releasing tension in the hips, groins, and gluteal region.

Ustrasana

Camel Pose

oosh-TRAHS-anna

ustra = camel

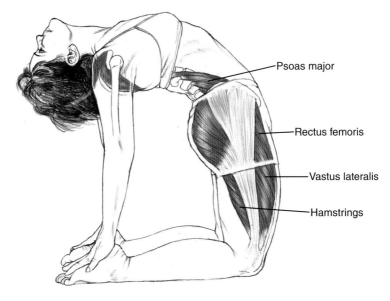

- Psoas major
- Rectus femoris
- Vastus lateralis
- Hamstrings

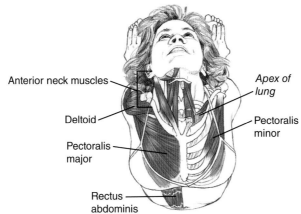

- Anterior neck muscles
- Deltoid
- Pectoralis major
- Apex of lung
- Pectoralis minor
- Rectus abdominis

Classification

Symmetrical kneeling backward-bending pose

Skeletal joint actions		
Spine	**Upper limbs**	**Lower limbs**
Extension	Scapular adduction and downward rotation, shoulder extension and adduction, elbow extension	SI joint counternutation, hip extension and adduction, knee flexion, ankle plantar flexion

Muscular joint actions

Spine

Concentric contraction	Eccentric contraction	Passively lengthening
To extend spine (though most of action of extension is caused by gravity): Spinal extensors	**To prevent overmobilization of lumbar spine:** Psoas minor, abdominal muscles **To resist hyperextension in cervical spine as head extends:** Anterior neck muscles	Psoas major

Upper limbs

Concentric contraction		Passively lengthening
To adduct, elevate, and downwardly rotate scapula: Rhomboids, levator scapulae **To stabilize shoulder joint and prevent protraction of head of humerus:** Rotator cuff	**To extend and adduct shoulder joint:** Triceps brachii (long head), teres major, posterior deltoid **To extend elbow:** Triceps brachii	Pectoralis major and minor, biceps brachii, coracobrachialis

Lower limbs

Concentric contraction	Eccentric contraction
To extend, adduct, and internally rotate hip: Hamstrings, adductor magnus, gluteus maximus	**To resist hip extension and knee flexion:** Rectus femoris **To resist knee flexion:** Articularis genu, vastii

Notes

Gravity is pulling the torso into the back bend, which is checked by the arm action and the eccentric action of the spinal flexors.

In the cervical spine, the anterior neck muscles are eccentrically active, but the sternocleidomastoid should not be active to avoid the base of the skull being pulled into the atlas and axis.

Internal rotation of the legs will help stabilize the SI joint by encouraging the front of this joint to align.

It can be very challenging to find a healthy extension of the spine at the base of the neck or the top of the thoracic spine. It helps to focus on releasing the sternocleidomastoid using the eccentric strength of the deeper anterior neck muscles to stabilize the weight of the head. Ustrasana can be an intense mobilization for the digestive system, especially the esophagus.

Breathing

In ustrasana, the thoracic structures are maintained in an inhalation position, and the abdominal wall is lengthened. This results in a decreased ability of the body to breathe "normally." The trick is to find support from the deeper musculature so that the more superficial efforts can quiet down. Then it's possible to notice an interesting relationship between the deepest layer of superficial neck muscles (scalenes) and the breath movement in the apex of the lungs, which are suspended from the inner scalene muscles.

Eka Pada Rajakapotasana

One-Legged Royal Pigeon Pose

eh-KAH pah-DAH rah-JAH-cop-poh-TAHS-anna

eka = one; *pada* = foot, leg; *raja* = king, royal; *kapota* = dove, pigeon

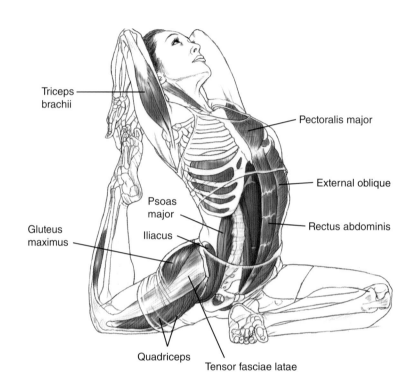

Triceps brachii

Pectoralis major

External oblique

Psoas major

Rectus abdominis

Gluteus maximus

Iliacus

Quadriceps

Tensor fasciae latae

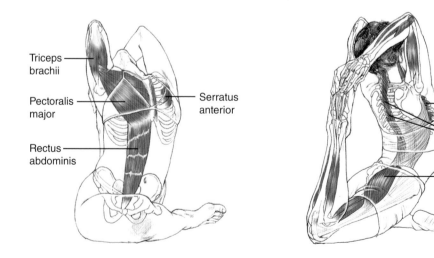

Triceps brachii

Pectoralis major

Rectus abdominis

Serratus anterior

Serratus anterior

Spinal extensors

Gluteus maximus

Classification

Asymmetrical kneeling backward-bending pose

Skeletal joint actions

Spine	Upper limbs	Lower limbs	
		Front leg	Back leg
Extension	Scapular upward rotation, abduction, and elevation; shoulder flexion, adduction, and external rotation; forearm supination; hand and finger flexion	SI joint nutation, hip flexion and external rotation, knee flexion, ankle plantar flexion, foot supination	SI joint counternutation; hip extension, internal rotation, and adduction; knee flexion; ankle plantar flexion

Muscular joint actions

Spine

Concentric contraction		Eccentric contraction
To extend spine: Spinal extensors	To neutralize twist from position of back leg: Internal oblique (front leg side); external oblique (back leg side)	To prevent hyperextension at lumbar spine: Psoas minor, abdominal muscles

Upper limbs

Concentric contraction	
To abduct, upwardly rotate, and elevate scapula: Serratus anterior, upper trapezius To stabilize, flex, and adduct shoulder joint: Rotator cuff, pectoralis major (upper fibers), anterior deltoid, biceps brachii (short head)	To rotate forearm and grasp foot: Supinator and flexors of hand and fingers

Lower limbs

Front leg	Back leg	
Eccentric contraction	Concentric contraction	Passively lengthening
To resist hip flexion: Hamstrings, piriformis, obturator internus, superior and inferior gemellus	To create hip extension and knee flexion: Hamstrings To create hip extension, internal rotation, and adduction: Adductor magnus	Iliacus, psoas major, rectus femoris

(continued)

Notes

It is important not to collapse into this pose. The pelvic floor, hamstrings, and gluteals should act eccentrically to distribute the weight created by the force of gravity through the whole base of the pose rather than drop right into the hamstring attachment or knee joint.

As with all poses, and more so with complex ones, a wide variety of experiences are available, depending on each person's strength, balance, and range of motion.

This pose is categorized as a kneeling pose because that is the starting position, but the base of support is not actually kneeling. This asana has a unique base of support: the back surface of the front leg and the front surface of the back leg. This same base, with the knee joints extended, would almost be hanumanasana (page 156).

Even though the front leg is externally rotated, this pose still requires a great deal of length in muscles of external rotation such as the piriformis, obturator internus, and superior and inferior gemellus. This is because these muscles are also hip extensors and abductors, and the actions in the front leg are hip flexion and adduction—the more adducted the front leg is, the more sensation will probably be felt in those muscles.

When the knee is more extended in the front leg (toward 90 degrees of flexion), the rotation at the hip is greatly intensified. This action puts more pressure into the knee, especially if there is restriction in the hip joint, and the knee is much more vulnerable to twisting forces when at 90 degrees. The action in the feet and ankles can help to stabilize and protect the knee.

Eka Pada Rajakapotasana Variation

Folded Forward

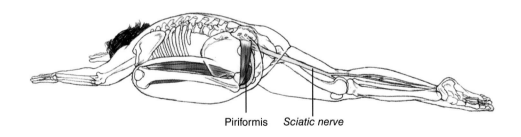

Piriformis   *Sciatic nerve*

Notes

This variation intensifies the actions in the hamstrings and other hip extensors (such as the piriformis) of the front leg because of deeper hip flexion and more body weight over the front leg. At the same time, it diminishes the actions in the back hip and in the spine.

This position is frequently used to "stretch" the piriformis muscle and the sciatic nerve. When sciatic pain exists, however, it is not necessarily useful to stretch the sciatic nerve, and the piriformis is not always responsible for sciatic pain. It may indeed be true that doing this asana often helps relieve this pain, but it's more likely that the mobilization of the hips and pelvis and the effects on all the muscles of the lower body are responsible.

The following illustrations show the relationship of the sciatic nerve to the piriformis muscle in:

1. neutral hip position (figure *a*);
2. external rotation and abduction, which actually shorten the piriformis (figure *b*);
3. hip flexion, which begins the lengthening of the piriformis and other external rotators (figure *c*);
4. and hip flexion combined with adduction, which puts the piriformis into maximal length, along with the sciatic nerve (figure *d*).

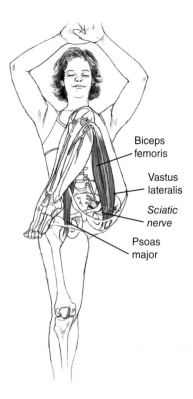

Biceps femoris

Vastus lateralis

Sciatic nerve

Psoas major

Folded-forward variation.

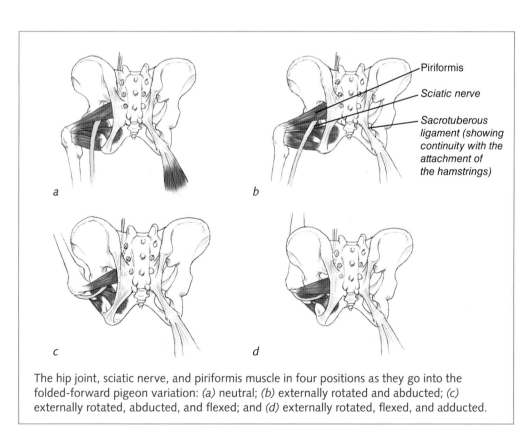

a

b

Piriformis

Sciatic nerve

Sacrotuberous ligament (showing continuity with the attachment of the hamstrings)

c

d

The hip joint, sciatic nerve, and piriformis muscle in four positions as they go into the folded-forward pigeon variation: *(a)* neutral; *(b)* externally rotated and abducted; *(c)* externally rotated, abducted, and flexed; and *(d)* externally rotated, flexed, and adducted.

Parighasana
Gate-Latch Pose

par-ee-GOSS-anna

parigha = an iron bar used for locking a gate

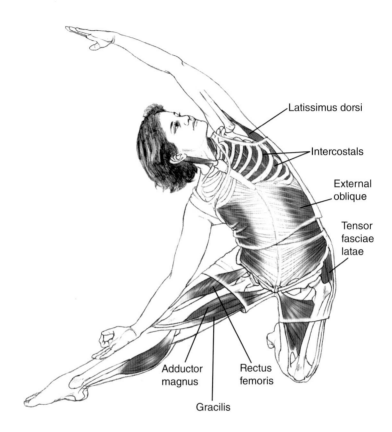

Latissimus dorsi

Intercostals

External oblique

Tensor fasciae latae

Adductor magnus

Rectus femoris

Gracilis

Classification

Asymmetrical kneeling side-bending pose

Skeletal joint actions

Spine	Upper limbs		Lower limbs	
	Top arm	Lower arm	Kneeling leg	Extended leg
Lateral flexion, cervical rotation and extension	Scapular upward rotation and elevation, shoulder abduction, elbow extension	Shoulder abduction, forearm supination	Hip extension and adduction, knee flexion, ankle dorsiflexion	Hip flexion, external rotation, and abduction; knee extension; ankle plantar flexion

Muscular joint actions

Spine

Concentric contraction	Eccentric contraction
To orient torso to front:	**To resist falling into gravity:**
Internal oblique (flexed leg side); external oblique (extended leg side)	External oblique, quadratus lumborum (flexed leg side)

Upper limbs

Upper arm

Concentric contraction	Eccentric contraction
To upwardly rotate, abduct, and elevate scapula:	**To extend arm overhead without falling into gravity:**
Serratus anterior	Teres major, latissimus dorsi
To stabilize shoulder joint:	
Rotator cuff	
To extend elbow:	
Triceps brachii, anconeus	

Lower limbs

Extended leg		Kneeling leg		
Concentric contraction	Eccentric contraction	Concentric contraction	Eccentric contraction	Passively lengthening
To rotate and abduct leg: Sartorius, piriformis, superior and inferior gemellus, obturator internus	**To keep from collapsing into hip:** Hamstrings	**To extend, adduct, and internally rotate hip:** Hamstrings, adductor magnus, gluteus maximus	**To resist hip extension and knee flexion:** Rectus femoris **To resist knee flexion:** Articularis genu, vastii	Gluteus medius and minimus, tensor fasciae latae

(continued)

Notes

Rotation is automatic with side bending in the spine because of both the shape of the articular facets in the vertebrae and the spiral pathways of the muscles. To keep the action pure lateral flexion, the upper and lower ribs need to counterrotate in relation to each other. In this case, the upper ribs rotate posteriorly and the lower ribs rotate anteriorly. To achieve this, the internal obliques on the upper side and the external obliques on the lower side are recruited.

Also, if tightness exists in the outside of the standing leg hip joint (in the tensor fasciae latae, gluteus medius, or gluteus minimus), then that hip will try to flex rather than stay purely adducted. The standing leg should maintain hip extension (via the adductor magnus and hamstrings) to prevent this.

When there is tightness in the latissimus dorsi, lifting the arm overhead can push the rib cage forward (compressing the floating ribs and inhibiting breath in general) or pull the scapula downward even as the arm is lifting, potentially creating impingement of the biceps brachii tendon or supraspinatus at the acromion process.

Breathing

Which side of the diaphragm moves more in this pose—the upper, lengthened side or the lower, compressed side? Is the answer the same for both sides of your body? Explore.

Simhasana

Lion Pose

sim-HAHS-anna

simha = lion

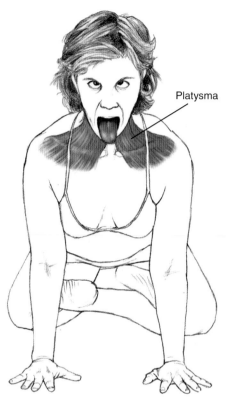

Platysma

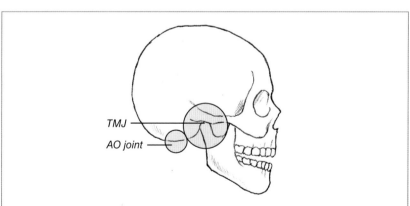

The temporomandibular joint (TMJ) represents the center of gravity of the skull, while the atlanto-occipital joint (AO joint) is its base of support.

Classification

Symmetrical kneeling pose

(continued)

Skeletal joint actions

Spine

Atlanto-occipital joint flexion, neutral spine, adduction and elevation of eyeballs

Notes

The lengthening activation of the tongue lifts the hyoid bone; activates the digestive system; and activates the hyoid muscles, sternum, rectus abdominis, pubic bone, and pelvic floor.

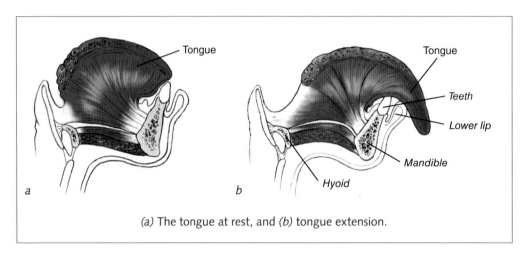

(a) The tongue at rest, and *(b)* tongue extension.

A strong exhalation (lion's roar) activates the three diaphragms: thoracic, pelvic, and vocal. The platysma muscle can also be contracted in simhasana. The superior and medial rectus muscles of the eyes both contract to direct the gaze inward and upward.

Simhasana stimulates and releases a host of often overlooked muscles. The tongue and jaw can be thought of as the front of the neck, and cervical tension can frequently be related to tightness in these structures. Additionally, the platysma (the flat, thin, rectangular muscle that covers the front of the throat) can be tonified during simhasana. Aside from the cosmetic advantages (a weak platysma is associated with wrinkly throat skin), consciously contracting this muscle increases the ability to relax it during inspiratory efforts.

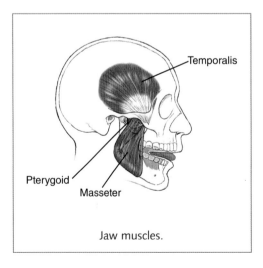

Jaw muscles.

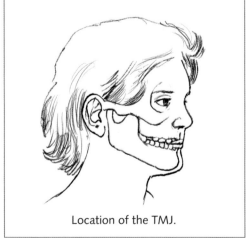

Location of the TMJ.

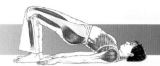
Supine means lying in a faceup position. It is the opposite of prone, which is lying face down. Similarly, supination means to turn a hand, foot, or limb upward, whereas pronation refers to turning them downward.

Both words originate from Latin: *Supinus* means leaning backward, and *pronus* means leaning forward. Interestingly, this is the reverse of the usual movement from each position. From a supine position, flexion in the spine and limbs is generally what moves the body into space; from a prone position, it is extension in the spine or limbs.

Moving into postures from a supine position generally engages the anterior musculature of the body, which is why many abdominal strengthening exercises start in this position.

Just as tadasana (page 72) is a quintessential standing position, savasana (page 182) is a fundamental supine position. In savasana, the back surface of the body is almost completely in contact with the support of the floor. There is nowhere to fall, so the postural muscles can relax from their constant dance with gravity.

Savasana has the lowest center of gravity possible and is a starting point for all the supine poses. It is also the position in which those asanas usually end. Because very little effort is required to stabilize the body while it is supine, poses that evolve from here are by definition mostly langhana and become more brhmana (see page 20) as the center of gravity is raised higher.

Savasana

Corpse Pose

shah-VAHS-anna

sava = corpse

This pose is also referred to as the death pose, or mrtasana (mrit-TAHS-anna). *Mrta* means death.

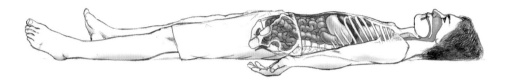

Classification

Symmetrical supine pose

Notes

Savasana is said to be the easiest asana to perform but the hardest to master. Whatever gymnastic demands the other asanas may make on your balance, strength, or flexibility, the challenge of maintaining awareness without effort or exertion is perhaps the most revealing exploration of body–mind integration we can engage in.

In savasana, the structures that are in full, weight-bearing contact with the floor exhibit the primary curves of the body (see page 37 of chapter 2). These include the posterior surfaces of the heels, calves, thighs, buttocks, rib cage, thoracic spine, scapulae, and skull.

The structures that are off the floor mirror the secondary curves of the body, specifically the hollows of the back of the ankles, knee joints, lumbar region, and cervical spine.

The points of contact of the arms vary widely from person to person, and the arms can be arranged in a variety of positions.

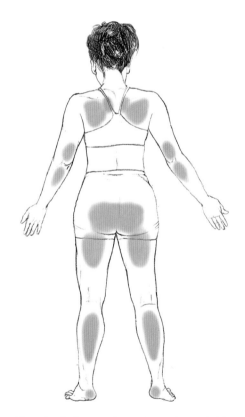

Blue shaded areas show the major weight-bearing structures, including most primary curves.

Symmetry

Often in savasana the limbs are carefully placed to be symmetrical when viewed from the outside. This can conflict with the body's kinesthetic (proprioceptive) feedback because what *looks* symmetrical is not what always *feels* symmetrical. We can negotiate this contrast in inner and outer experience in a variety of ways.

It can sometimes be useful to align the structures as symmetrically as possible and then see if you can receive the kinesthetic feedback of the sensations of asymmetry without needing to respond. Perhaps your proprioceptors can even adapt to this new information and redefine your perception of neutral.

Alternatively, it can also be valuable to organize more from the inside and seek inner comfort and quiet, regardless of how asymmetrically the limbs are arranged. We can find balance without being symmetrical, which is a valuable distinction for everyone to recognize because none of our internal structures are symmetrical. Nevertheless, they all have the ability to find balance and harmony. Because all human bodies are inherently asymmetrical, a certain amount of surrender to this fact is necessary to achieve a deep state of emotional and physical integration.

Breathing

A deep state of quiet consciousness is quite different from sleep, which is a common experience in this pose. In savasana, the body is completely at rest and its metabolism is freed of the demands of contending with gravity, making it possible to practice the most difficult breathing exercise of all: the act of being fully aware of—but not controlling—the breath's movements.

Usually, when you are aware of your breathing, in some way you alter its natural rhythm. When you are not aware of the breath, it is driven by a combination of autonomic impulses and unconscious habit. The juxtaposition of active awareness and surrender to the breath's natural movements makes possible the powerful realization that true surrender is an act of will.

Apanasana

Apana Pose, Wind Release Pose

ap-an-AHS-anna

apana = the vital air that eliminates waste from the system

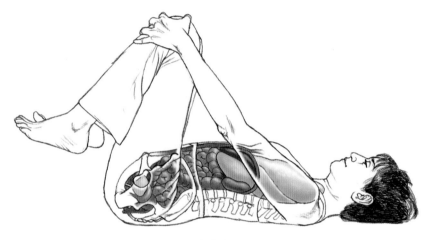

Inhalation.

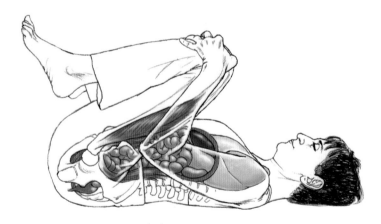

Exhalation.

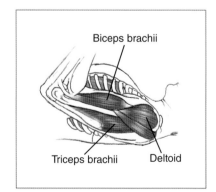

Biceps brachii

Triceps brachii

Deltoid

Classification

Symmetrical supine forward-bending vinyasa

Notes

Apanasana is one of the key tools of therapeutic yoga because it is a simple and accessible practice that directly links breath and body movement. In this simple vinyasa, or sequence, the hands are on the knees, and with the inhale the legs move away from the body. With the exhale the legs move toward the body. This movement can be created in a variety of ways: through the very gentle movement of the breath, a simple movement of the limbs, or a more vigorous movement of the spine.

Breathing

Apanasana stimulates the upward release of the diaphragm on the exhalation as the knees are drawn into the body either by actively using the abdominal and hip flexor muscles or by using the arms to pump the thighs against the abdomen and leaving the abdominals and hip flexors passive.

Low-back tension can be the result of tension in the diaphragm. Performing apanasana is a simple and effective way of helping the lower spine by mobilizing the contents of the abdomen and creating more diaphragmatic space for the abdominal muscles to create postural support.

Taken together, dwi pada pitham (page 188) and apanasana constitute a powerful pair of counterposing movements that can facilitate profound changes and healing.

Setu Bandhasana

Bridge Pose

SET-too bahn-DAHS-anna

setu = dam, dike, bridge; *bandha* = lock; *setubandha* = the forming of a causeway or bridge; dam, bridge

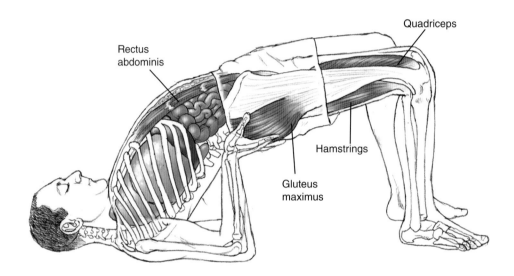

Classification

Symmetrical supine inverted pose

Skeletal joint actions		
Spine	**Upper limbs**	**Lower limbs**
Cervical and upper thoracic flexion, lower thoracic and lumbar extension	Scapular adduction, downward rotation, and elevation; shoulder extension and adduction; elbow flexion; forearm supination; wrist dorsiflexion	SI joint counternutation, hip extension, knee extension, ankle dorsiflexion

Muscular joint actions

Spine

Concentric contraction	Eccentric contraction
To extend lower thoracic and lumbar spine:	**To resist lumbar hyperextension:**
Spinal extensors	Psoas minor, abdominal muscles

Upper limbs

Concentric contraction	Eccentric contraction
To adduct, elevate, and downwardly rotate scapula:	**To receive and support weight of pelvis:**
Rhomboids, levator scapulae	Flexors of wrist and hand
To stabilize shoulder joint and prevent protraction of head of humerus:	
Rotator cuff	
To extend and adduct shoulder joint:	
Triceps brachii (long head), teres major, posterior deltoid	
To flex elbow and supinate forearm:	
Biceps brachii, brachialis	

Lower limbs

Concentric contraction	Passively lengthening
To extend hip:	Psoas major, iliacus
Hamstrings, gluteus maximus	
To extend, adduct, and internally rotate hip:	
Adductor magnus, gracilis	
To extend knee:	
Articularis genu, vastii	

Notes

It can be a challenge to find full hip extension in this pose without also adducting or externally rotating at the hip joints. If the hamstrings and adductor magnus are not strong enough, the gluteus maximus may do too much and pull the legs into external rotation, the other adductors (such as the pectineus) may activate to bring the knees together but also flex the hips, or the rectus femoris may work to extend the knees but interfere with the ability to extend the hips.

Spinal extensors (especially lumbar) may be useful, but too much lumbar extension is not helpful because it may limit hip extension by putting tension on the psoas complex.

While the final position of the knees is actually a flexed shape, the action of coming into the pose is one of extension because it is moving from more flexion to less flexion.

The elevation of the scapulae moves the shoulder blades into the floor, which then lifts the rib cage away from the floor. It is important that the scapulae are not depressed or pulled down the back in this position, because that action moves the scapulae away from the cervical spine, leaving the flexed neck to bear the weight of the upper body.

(continued)

The action in the arms is also the foundation for salamba sarvangasana (page 190) and viparita karani (page 196); the action in the hips and legs is the same as for lifting into urdhva dhanurasana (page 249).

All in all, considering the many muscle actions that must be balanced for this pose to work, sustaining this basic posture actually requires a high degree of coordination.

Breathing

This position offers the opportunity to experience all three bandhas: the lower abdominal action of mula bandha, the opening at the base of the rib cage (supported by the hand position) of uddiyana bandha, and the chin lock associated with cervical flexion known as jalandhara bandha.

Setu Bandhasana Variation

Dwi Pada Pitham
Two-Legged Table
dvee PA-da PEET-ham
dwi = two; *pada* = feet; *pitham* = stool, seat, chair, bench

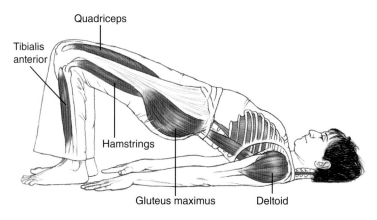
Inhalation.

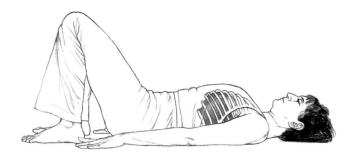
Exhalation.

Classification

Symmetrical supine vinyasa

Notes

Except for the arm position, the muscular, spinal, and joint actions of this pose are virtually identical to those of setu bandhasana. The main difference between setu bandhasana and dwi pada pitham is that dwi pada pitham is a vinyasa, a dynamic movement that is coordinated with the inhalation and exhalation.

This simple yet versatile practice can be used in a variety of ways to release tension from the spine and breathing structures, as well as to help balance the leg and hip actions that support similar poses, such as setu bandhasana and urdhva dhanurasana (page 249).

Breathing

The lifting movement is typically done on the inhalation and the lowering on the exhalation, but this pattern can be changed to produce various effects. For example, the three bandhas can be very easily activated simply by doing the lowering movement while suspending the breath at the end of an exhale (bhaya kumbaka). Lowering the spine while using bhaya kumbhaka creates a natural lifting of the pelvic floor and abdominal contents toward the zone of lowered pressure in the thoracic cavity. The subsequent inhalation can create a dramatic downward release of the pelvic floor and a noticeable sense of relaxation in this often tense region.

Salamba Sarvangasana

Supported Shoulder Stand

sah-LOM-bah sar-van-GAHS-anna

salamba = with support (*sa* = with, *alamba* = support); *sarva* = all; *anga* = limb

The term *salamba* distinguishes this variation of the shoulder stand from the unsupported (niralamba) version.

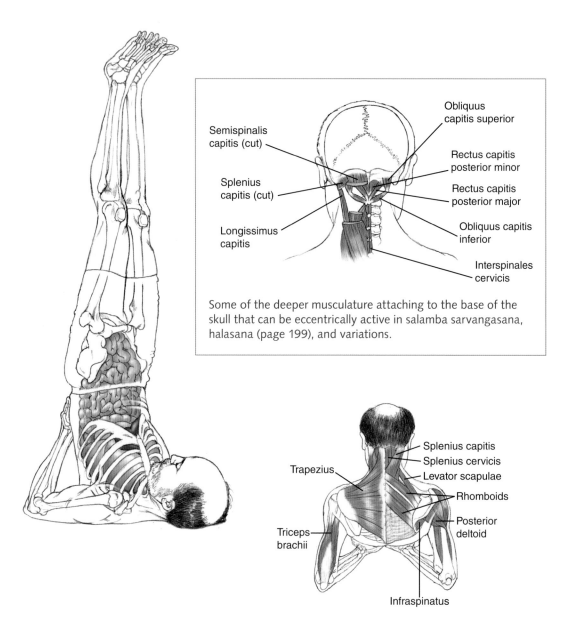

Some of the deeper musculature attaching to the base of the skull that can be eccentrically active in salamba sarvangasana, halasana (page 199), and variations.

Classification

Symmetrical supine inverted pose

Skeletal joint actions

Spine	Upper limbs	Lower limbs
Cervical and upper thoracic flexion, lower thoracic and lumbar extension	Scapular adduction, downward rotation, and elevation; shoulder extension and adduction; elbow flexion; forearm supination; wrist dorsiflexion	Hip extension and adduction, knee extension, ankle dorsiflexion

Muscular joint actions

Spine

	Eccentric contraction
To calibrate concentric and eccentric contractions to support spine: Spinal extensors and flexors	**To resist flexion from weight of body:** Cervical spinal extensors

Upper limbs

Concentric contraction

To adduct, elevate, and downwardly rotate scapula: Rhomboids, levator scapulae	**To extend and adduct shoulder joint:** Triceps brachii (long head), teres major, posterior deltoid
To stabilize shoulder joint and prevent protraction of head of humerus: Rotator cuff	**To flex elbow and supinate forearm:** Biceps brachii, brachialis
	To support rib cage: Flexors of wrist and hand

Lower limbs

Concentric contraction

To resist leg falling toward face: Hamstrings, gluteus maximus	**To extend knee:** Vastii
To extend, adduct, and internally rotate hip: Adductor magnus, gracilis	

(continued)

Notes

The foundation of this pose, as in setu bandhasana (page 186), is the shoulder girdle (not the neck). To truly be a shoulder stand, the muscles that elevate, adduct, and downwardly rotate the scapulae must be strong enough to keep the scapulae in that position despite the weight of the entire body resting on them. When preparing for this pose, it is essential that the scapulae find elevation along with the other actions; if the scapulae are depressed, the cervical spine receives the weight of the whole body in a flexed position, which makes it very vulnerable to injury.

Entering the pose from halasana (page 199) is more demanding on the extensors of the spine, especially the thoracic spine, because they are in an elongated position before contracting. Entering from setu bandhasana is more demanding on the extensors of the shoulder joints and the flexors of the spine (the psoas and abdominal muscles).

From the perspective of the muscles of the spine and abdomen, being in this pose is less challenging than getting into it. However, remaining in the pose is more challenging for the muscles of the scapulae, because they are bearing the static load of the body.

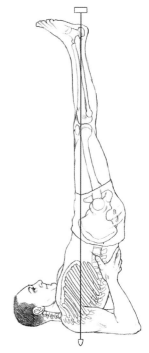

Center line of gravity passing through the base of support.

Breathing

The more mobility that exists in the scapulae (or the less resistance from other muscles of the thorax), the less compromised the breath is in this position. This pose takes a tremendous amount of both flexibility and strength in the entire shoulder girdle. Without the integrity of the shoulder girdle, the weight collapses down into the thorax and the diaphragm becomes obstructed.

Keeping the base of the rib cage open allows the diaphragm and abdominal viscera to shift effectively toward the head so the full benefits of inversion can occur.

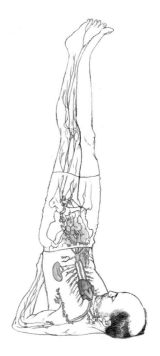

Lymph drainage in shoulder stand.

192

Niralamba Sarvangasana
Unsupported (No-Arm) Shoulder Stand

neera-LOM-bah sar-van-GAHS-anna

niralamba = no support, independent, self-supported; *sarva* = all; *anga* = limb

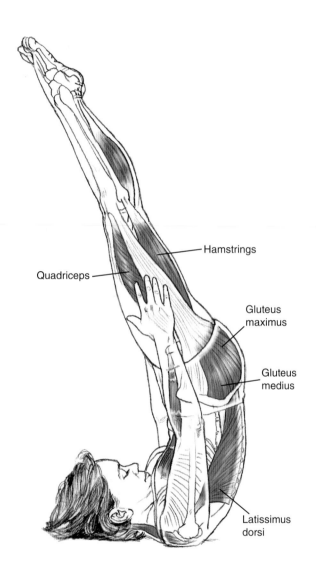

Hamstrings

Quadriceps

Gluteus maximus

Gluteus medius

Latissimus dorsi

Classification

Symmetrical supine inverted pose

(continued)

Skeletal joint actions

Spine	Upper limbs	Lower limbs
Cervical and upper thoracic flexion, lower thoracic and lumbar extension	Scapular adduction, upward rotation, and elevation; shoulder adduction; elbow extension; forearm pronation	Hip extension and adduction, knee extension, ankle dorsiflexion

Muscular joint actions

Spine

To calibrate concentric and eccentric contractions to support spine: Spinal extensors and flexors	*Eccentric contraction* **To resist flexion from weight of body:** Cervical spinal extensors

Upper limbs

Concentric contraction

To adduct, elevate, and upwardly rotate scapula: Trapezius, levator scapulae	**To stabilize shoulder joint and prevent protraction of head of humerus:** Rotator cuff
To upwardly rotate scapula: Serratus anterior	**To adduct shoulder and extend elbow:** Triceps brachii
To flex and adduct shoulder against pull of gravity: Teres minor, coracobrachialis	

Lower limbs

Concentric contraction

To resist leg falling toward face: Hamstrings, gluteus maximus	**To extend, adduct, and internally rotate hip:** Adductor magnus, gracilis **To extend knee:** Vastii

Notes

In this pose, the scapulae are elevated, adducted, and slightly upwardly rotated; without the levering action of the arms, this calls on the muscles that move the scapulae on the rib cage to work strongly. It might feel like contradictory actions to perform adduction, elevation, and upward rotation simultaneously. It is indeed possible and in fact necessary in this pose in order to protect the neck. If the scapulae are not maintained in adduction, the weight of the body falls into the spine; if the scapulae do not upwardly rotate, the arms are challenged in being alongside the body. The scapulae are positioned in neutral rotation as they extend to the knees, but the action that gets them there is upward rotation as they come from the downward rotation of niralamba sarvangasana.

The upper fibers of the psoas major and abdominal muscles are very strongly engaged here to maintain the spinal flexion in the thoracic spine. In addition, more lumbar flexion occurs to bring the legs farther overhead and counterbalance the pull of gravity. Resisting this tendency toward lumbar flexion makes the spinal flexors work much harder eccentrically against the body weight's tendency to roll down to the floor.

In this balancing act between spinal flexors and extensors, imbalances that are usually imperceptible show up because the arms aren't available to leverage symmetry. When these torques appear, they make this pose that much more challenging to balance.

Breathing

In niralamba sarvangasana, the intense action in the torso's flexor and extensor groups creates quite a challenge to the shape change of breathing. Because this is a challenging balance pose that requires a lot of stabilizing action in the abdominal and thoracic musculature, any attempt at deep breathing will destabilize the pose even as the full-body activation of these major muscle groups creates a demand for significant oxygenation.

Efficiency—finding the minimum amount of effort necessary to maintain the position—allows the limited breath movements to supply just enough energy to sustain the pose.

Viparita Karani

Inverted Pose

vip-par-ee-tah car-AHN-ee

viparita = turned around, reversed, inverted; *karani* = doing, making, action

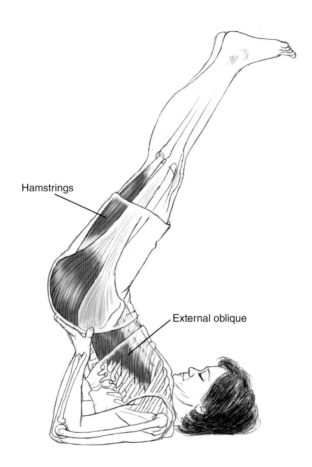

Hamstrings

External oblique

Classification

Symmetrical supine inverted pose

Skeletal joint actions

Spine	Upper limbs	Lower limbs
Cervical and upper thoracic flexion, lower thoracic and lumbar extension	Scapular adduction, downward rotation, and elevation; shoulder extension and adduction; elbow flexion; forearm supination; wrist dorsiflexion	Hip flexion and adduction, knee extension, ankle dorsiflexion

Muscular joint actions

Spine

Concentric contraction	Eccentric contraction
To extend lower thoracic spine: Spinal extensors	**To resist lumbar hyperextension and counter weight of leg:** Psoas major and minor, abdominal muscles

Upper limbs

Concentric contraction	Eccentric contraction
To adduct, elevate, and downwardly rotate scapula: Rhomboids, levator scapulae **To stabilize shoulder joint and prevent protraction of head of humerus:** Rotator cuff **To extend and adduct shoulder joint:** Triceps brachii (long head), teres major, posterior deltoid **To flex elbow and supinate forearm:** Biceps brachii, brachialis	**To receive and support weight of pelvis:** Flexors of wrist and hand

Lower limbs

Concentric contraction	Eccentric contraction
To extend knee: Vastii	**To resist leg falling toward face:** Hamstrings, gluteus maximus **To extend, adduct, and internally rotate hip:** Adductor magnus, gracilis

(continued)

197

Notes

In salamaba sarvangasana (page 190), the erector muscles of the spine are more active than in viparita karani. In the lifted version of viparita karani, the abdominal muscles play a greater role than the spinal muscles to keep the pelvis from collapsing onto the hands—because of the flexion of the hips, the weight of the legs falls in such a way that the weight of the pelvis is falling backward toward further extension in the spine.

In viparita karani, the abdominal muscles are strongly active in eccentric contraction. If they do not have the ability to modulate their lengthening, the weight of the pelvis collapses onto the hands or wrists. Practicing the ability to enter and leave this pose can help with other actions that require abdominal eccentric control, such as dropping the legs over into urdhva dhanurasana (page 249) from a headstand or handstand, controlling vrksasana (page 86), dropping back into urdhva dhanurasana from tadasana (page 72), and so forth.

Body proportions and individual differences in weight distribution between the upper and lower body greatly affect the

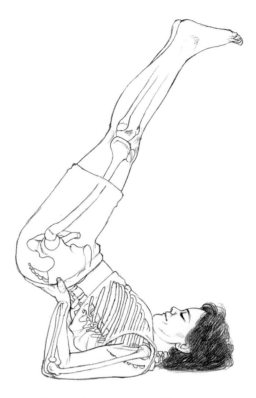

Dropped version of viparita karani.

experience of this pose. A prime example is how challenging controlling the movement into this pose can be for women because of the greater proportion of weight in their lower bodies and the generally greater flexibility of their spines.

Breathing

The inverted nature of viparita karani produces the cleansing, eliminative effects associated with the upward movement of apana. The supported versions of this pose are a valuable staple of restorative yoga practice.

Halasana

Plow Pose

hah-LAHS-anna

hala = plow

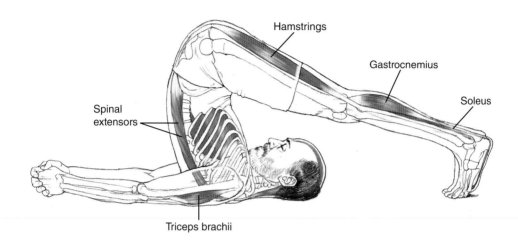

Hamstrings

Gastrocnemius

Soleus

Spinal
extensors

Triceps brachii

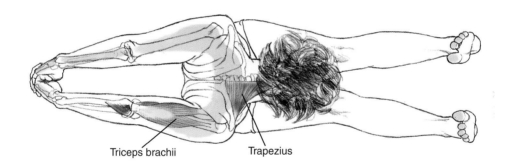

Triceps brachii

Trapezius

Classification

Symmetrical supine inverted forward-bending pose

Skeletal joint actions		
Spine	**Upper limbs**	**Lower limbs**
Flexion	Scapular adduction, downward rotation, and elevation; shoulder extension and adduction; elbow extension; forearm pronation; wrist extension; hand and finger flexion	SI joint nutation, hip flexion and adduction, knee extension, ankle dorsiflexion, toe extension

(continued)

Muscular joint actions		

Spine

Eccentric contraction

To resist flexion from weight of body:
Spinal extensors

Upper limbs

Concentric contraction

To adduct, elevate, and downwardly rotate scapula: Rhomboids, levator scapulae	**To extend and adduct shoulder joint:** Triceps brachii (long head), teres major, posterior deltoid
To stabilize shoulder joint and prevent protraction of head of humerus: Rotator cuff	**To extend elbow:** Triceps brachii
	To clasp hands: Flexors of hand and fingers

Lower limbs

Concentric contraction	*Eccentric contraction*	*Passively lengthening*
To extend knee: Vastii	**To maintain alignment of legs:** Hamstrings, adductor magnus, gracilis	Gastrocnemius, soleus
To dorsiflex ankle and tuck toes under: Tibialis anterior, toe extensors		

Notes

This pose has many variations: spine more or less extended, arms overhead, or hands on the back as in salamba sarvangasana (page 190). Some of these variations put more pressure into the spine than others. For example, when the arms reach overhead and clasp the toes, the scapulae upwardly rotate and move away from the spine, and weight falls into the upper spine. This variation can overmobilize the thoracic and cervical spine; there is potentially damaging pressure from the pushing action of the feet and, if the hamstrings and gluteals are tight, from the limited hip flexion forcing greater spinal flexion.

Because this pose can produce very intense flexion for the spine, especially the cervical region, it's more important to maintain the integrity of the scapulae and cervical and thoracic spine than to get the legs to the floor; support the legs if necessary to protect the neck.

Breathing

As in salamba sarvangasana, keeping the base of the rib cage open allows the diaphragm and abdominal viscera to shift effectively toward the head so the full benefits of inversion can occur. This can be much more of a challenge in this pose because the hip flexion tends to create more intra-abdominal pressure.

Halasana is a very good gauge of how freely you can breathe. It's one thing to have the range of motion and flexibility to get into the pose, but quite another to have the diaphragm and organs be free enough to remain there and breathe comfortably.

Karnapidasana

Ear-to-Knee Pose

KAR-na-peed-AHS-anna

karna = ear; *pidana* = squeeze, pressure

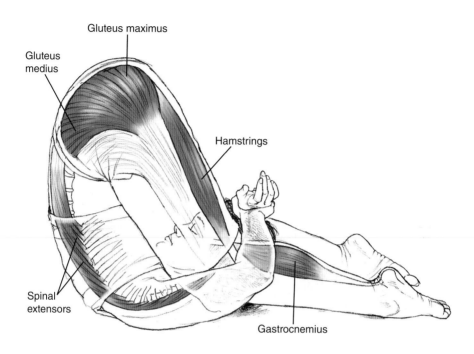

Gluteus maximus

Gluteus medius

Hamstrings

Spinal extensors

Gastrocnemius

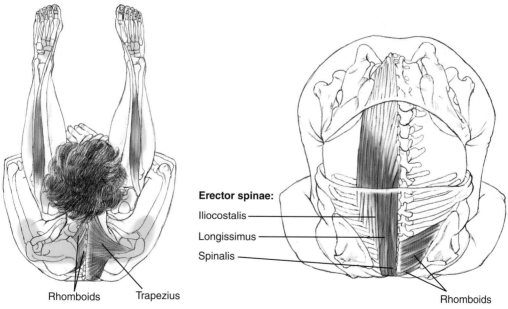

Rhomboids

Trapezius

Erector spinae:

Iliocostalis

Longissimus

Spinalis

Rhomboids

Classification

Symmetrical supine inverted forward-bending pose

(continued)

Skeletal joint actions		
Spine	**Upper limbs**	**Lower limbs**
Flexion	Scapular abduction and upward rotation, shoulder flexion, elbow flexion, hand and finger flexion	SI joint nutation, hip flexion, knee flexion, ankle plantar flexion

Muscular joint actions	
Spine	
Passively lengthening	
Spinal extensors	
Upper limbs	
Concentric contraction	*Passively lengthening*
To flex elbow:	Rhomboids, trapezius
Biceps brachii	
To clasp hands:	
Flexors of hand and fingers	
Lower limbs	
Passively lengthening	
Gluteus maximus	

Notes

Extensors of the spine should all lengthen evenly, ensuring that the opening is distributed along the whole spine. When the arms move overhead and the scapulae spread away from the spine, the weight bearing shifts to the spinous processes of the thoracic spine from the scapulae.

This variation can overstretch the thoracic and cervical spine due to the weight of the legs and pelvis, directing pressure into the vulnerable muscles of the neck and upper back.

This counterposes the shoulder action of sarvangasana (pages 190 and 193) because the spinal extension and scapular adduction of shoulder stand is reversed, so the muscles that were active are now lengthening. If the release is too passive, however, the muscles can be overlengthened.

Breathing

In this pose, the weight of the lower body is bearing down into the torso, which is in maximal flexion—this is basically an inverted, weight-bearing exhalation.

If the muscles are tense in this pose, even if the joints and muscles have enough flexibility, the breath is inhibited. This limitation soon results in the muscles' inability to fuel their activity; at this point, the asana should be exited.

Jathara Parivrtti

Belly Twist

JAT-hara par-ee-VRIT-ti

jathara = stomach, belly, abdomen, bowels, the interior of anything;
parivrtti = turning, rolling

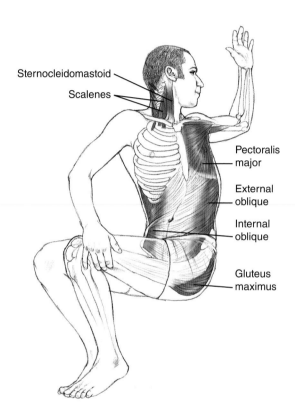

Classification

Asymmetrical supine twisting pose

Skeletal joint actions			
Spine	**Upper limbs**		**Lower limbs**
	Arm opposite leg	**Arm holding leg**	
Rotation	Scapular adduction, shoulder abduction and external rotation, elbow flexion	Scapular abduction, shoulder abduction and internal rotation, elbow flexion	Hip flexion, knee flexion

(continued)

Muscular joint actions

Spine

Passively lengthening

External oblique, intercostals, transversospinalis (top leg side); internal oblique, intercostals, oblique muscles of erector spinae (bottom leg side)

Upper limbs

Passively lengthening

Pectoralis major and minor, coracobrachialis, latissimus dorsi (arm opposite leg)

Lower limbs

Passively lengthening

Gluteus maximus, medius, and minimus; piriformis; superior and inferior gemellus; obturator internus (top leg)

Notes

To ensure that this twist is evenly distributed throughout the spine, it is important to maintain a neutral spine. This is a challenge with both knees bent because it's much easier to move into lumbar flexion to deepen the rotation. However, this might put excess pressure into the lumbar vertebrae and discs. If there is a lack of balanced mobility in the spine, excessive force can be directed into vulnerable spots such as the disc between T11 and T12 or the front of the shoulder joint.

Breathing

Because the body is supported by the floor and the main action is provided by gravity, the breathing and postural muscles are free to release in jathara parivrtti. The breath can thus be directed in various ways to achieve specific effects. For example, bringing the breath movements to the abdomen releases the tone in the abdominal wall and pelvic floor and assists in reducing extraneous muscle tension in the lumbar region. The opposite pattern of restraining the abdominal wall during the inhalation directs the action of the diaphragm into the thoracic structures, mobilizing the costovertebral joints. A similar effect can be achieved in the seated twists (see the discussion of ardha matsyendrasana on page 152 of chapter 7).

Jathara Parivrtti Variation

With Legs Extended

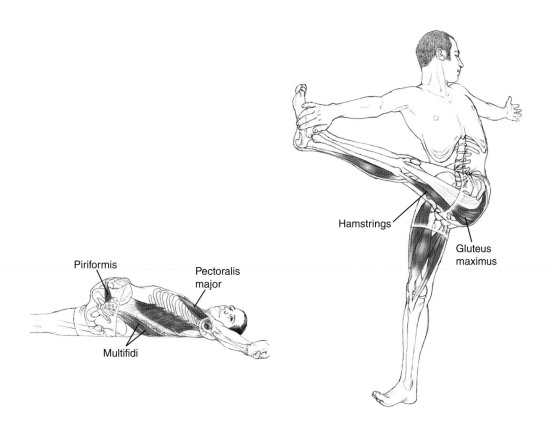

Piriformis

Pectoralis
major

Multifidi

Hamstrings

Gluteus
maximus

Notes

In this variation, the top leg's hamstrings are lengthening; tightness here can contribute to spinal flexion. The bottom leg's hamstrings are active and help counter spinal flexion with extensor action.

With the bottom leg extended, the top leg has more adduction and possibly more internal rotation, which leads to increased length in the iliotibial band; gluteus minimus, medius, and maximus; piriformis; superior and inferior gemellus; and obturator internus.

Matsyasana

Fish Pose

mots-YAHS-anna

matsya = fish

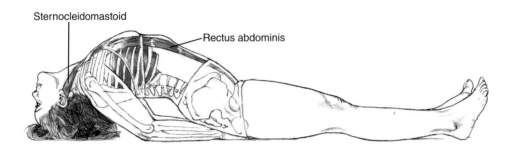

Sternocleidomastoid

Rectus abdominis

Classification

Symmetrical supine backward-bending pose

Skeletal joint actions		
Spine	**Upper limbs**	**Lower limbs**
Extension	Scapular downward rotation and adduction, shoulder extension and adduction, elbow flexion, forearm pronation	Hip flexion and adduction, knee extension

Spine

Concentric contraction	Eccentric contraction
To lift spine from floor in extension: Spinal extensors **To extend spine (and flex hip):** Psoas major	**To resist hyperextension in cervical and lumbar spine:** Anterior neck muscles, psoas minor, abdominal muscles

Upper limbs

Concentric contraction	Passively lengthening
To stabilize shoulder joint: Rotator cuff **To internally rotate, extend, and adduct arm at shoulder:** Latissimus dorsi **To extend shoulder joint and press hand into floor:** Triceps brachii **To adduct scapula:** Trapezius, rhomboids **To turn hand toward floor:** Pronator quadratus and teres	Coracobrachialis, pectoralis major and minor

Lower limbs

Concentric contraction	
To flex hip (and extend spine): Psoas major, iliacus **To ground leg:** Hamstrings	**To flex hip and extend knee:** Quadriceps

Notes

This pose can be done while focusing on using spinal extensors (which include the psoas major on the front of the spine) or supporting on the elbows. If the support of the elbows is used, there is less work in the muscles of the torso and perhaps more ease in breathing and more expansion.

If the pose is done while focusing on the muscles that extend the spine, the neck is better protected when lifting the arms off the floor. Variations can also be done with blocks under the spine and with the feet in baddha konasana (page 144) or padmasana (page 127).

This pose provides a great demonstration of the role of the psoas major in both hip flexion and spinal extension.

This pose is frequently used as an immediate counterpose to salamba sarvangasana (page 190) because it reverses the position of the cervical spine from extreme flexion to extreme extension. However, going from one static extreme to the other may not be the most beneficial way to compensate for the stresses of salamba sarvangasana. A more dynamic approach would be to gradually reverse the movement of the neck with simple vinyasas leading up to bhujangasana (page 212).

(continued)

Breathing

In matsyasana the chest is expanded, but not as maximally as in the more difficult arm-supported urdhva dhanurasana (page 249). As a result, there is still room for the inhaling action to further expand the rib cage, using the arms as leverage.

For a more calming effect—particularly if using matsyasana as a counterpose—focusing on gentle abdominal breathing can be quite useful.

Matsyasana Variation

With Arms and Legs Lifted

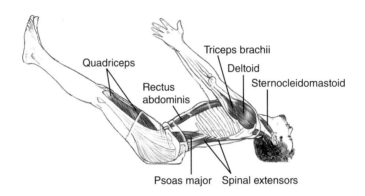

Notes

There is greatly increased action in the legs when lifted off the floor, especially in the psoas major, iliacus, and rectus femoris.

With the change in arm position, the coracobrachialis, no longer lengthening, is now working to flex and adduct the arm, as are the pectorals and anterior deltoid. The serratus anterior muscles are recruited to abduct the scapulae, and the triceps brachii are extending the elbows.

Anantasana

Reclining Vishnu Couch Pose

anan-TAHS-anna

ananta = endless, eternal (*anta* = end, *an* = without)

Ananta is also the name given to the mythical serpent that the god Vishnu reclines on like a couch.

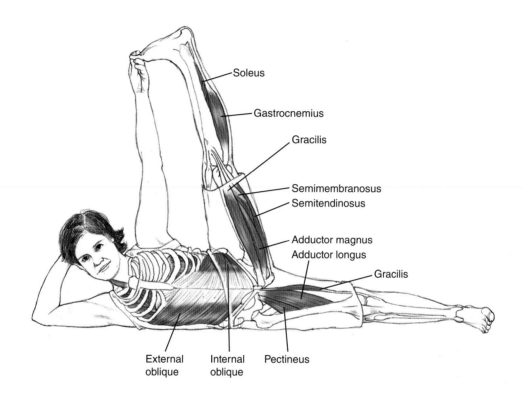

Classification

Asymmetrical side-lying balancing pose

Skeletal joint actions				
Spine	Upper limbs		Lower limbs	
	Top arm	Bottom arm	Top leg	Bottom leg
Lateral flexion	Shoulder abduction, elbow extension	Scapular upward rotation and elevation, shoulder flexion, elbow flexion	Hip flexion, abduction, and external rotation; knee extension	Neutral hip extension, knee extension

(continued)

Muscular joint actions		

Spine

Concentric contraction	Eccentric contraction	Passively lengthening
To create side bend:	**To stabilize curves of spine:**	Quadratus lumborum (bottom side)
Spinal extensors, internal and external oblique, quadratus lumborum (top side)	Spinal extensors, internal and external oblique (bottom side)	

Lower limbs

Top leg		Bottom leg
Concentric contraction	Passively lengthening	Concentric contraction
To externally rotate and abduct:	Hamstrings, adductor magnus, gastrocnemius, soleus	**To resist hip flexion:**
Gluteus medius and minimus (posterior fibers), piriformis, obturator internus, superior and inferior gemellus		Hamstrings
		To press lower leg into floor for stability:
To flex hip:		Gluteus medius and minimus
Psoas major, iliacus		
To flex hip and extend knee:		
Quadriceps		

Notes

When the leg is lifted, the pelvis and lower body often roll backward. The challenge is to find the balancing movement through the abductors and external rotators of the hip joint rather than through rotating the spine.

Breathing

Anantasana is one of the few true side-lying poses. In the side-lying position, the dome of the diaphragm closest to the floor moves cranially (toward the head), while the other dome moves caudally (toward the tail). This is due mainly to the effect of gravity on the abdominal organs, which are pulled toward the floor, taking the diaphragm with them. In addition, the lung closest to the floor (the dependent lung) becomes more supported and its tissue becomes more compliant, meaning that it's under less mechanical tension and responds more easily to the action of the diaphragm.

Consciously creating this asymmetry in the respiratory mechanism can be useful in breaking up deeply ingrained breathing habits. For example, this pose can be beneficial to people trying to change the habit of sleeping on only one side of the body.

Prone means lying in a facedown position. This is a position that everyone is able to maintain at birth, but adults often find uncomfortable. Sometimes the discomfort is a result of restricted movement in the neck and upper back that makes it hard to turn the head to the side. This position can also feel suffocating because the movement of the abdomen is inhibited by the weight of the body, and the back of the body has to be more mobile to breathe comfortably.

For some people this position has even more of a connotation of surrender than kneeling. In many religious traditions, placing the entire front surface of the body on the floor is known as a full prostration.

For others this position feels safer than being supine, because the vulnerable front body and organs are more protected.

From a prone position the easiest movement is extension in the spine and limbs, which uses the posterior musculature of the body. For this reason many back strengthening exercises begin in this position. Although the center of gravity in this position is close to the floor, poses that evolve from here are mostly brhmana (see page 20) because of the effort needed to lift the body away from the floor.

Bhujangasana
Cobra Pose

boo-jang-GAHS-anna

bhujanga = serpent (*bhuja* = arm, shoulder; *anga* = limb)

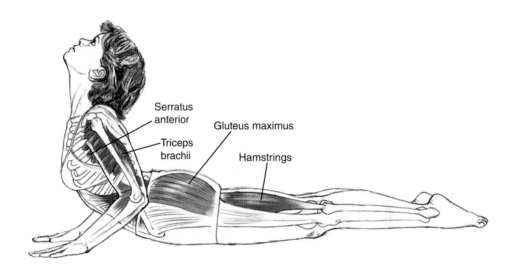

Serratus anterior

Triceps brachii

Gluteus maximus

Hamstrings

Classification

Symmetrical prone backward-bending pose

Skeletal joint actions		
Spine	**Upper limbs**	**Lower limbs**
Extension	Elbow extension, forearm pronation	SI joint counternutation, hip extension and adduction, knee extension, ankle plantar flexion

Muscular joint actions

Spine

Concentric contraction	Eccentric contraction
To extend spine:	**To prevent overmobilization of lumbar spine:**
Spinal extensors	Psoas minor, abdominal muscles
To extend thoracic spine and synergize with some of the spinal extensors, which it overlays:	
Serratus posterior superior	

Upper limbs

Concentric contraction	
To stabilize scapula on rib cage and translate push of arm into clavicle:	**To extend elbow:**
Serratus anterior	Triceps brachii
To stabilize shoulder joint:	**To pronate forearm:**
Rotator cuff	Pronator quadratus and teres

Lower limbs

Concentric contraction	
To extend, adduct, and internally rotate hip:	**To plantar flex ankle:**
Hamstrings, adductor magnus	Soleus
To extend knee:	
Vastii	

Notes

It is important to find the deeper intrinsic back muscles to do the action of spinal extension in this pose. Using the latissimus dorsi and other more superficial muscles affects the scapulae and rib cage and interferes with breathing by inhibiting the movement of the ribs.

In this pose, the serratus anterior is active to maintain a neutral position of the scapulae against the push of the arms. When the arms push, the shoulders don't elevate but the spine is lifted.

The latissimus dorsi are not helpful as extensors of the spine, because they create flexion of the upper back and internal rotation in the arms.

(continued)

Many people assume the legs should be passive in cobra, but numerous actions in the legs are required to keep the joints in alignment. The hamstrings, especially the semitendinosus and semimembranosus, extend the hips and maintain adduction and internal rotation. The extensor portion of the adductor magnus, along with the deep and medial fibers of the gluteus maximus, also extends the hips without externally rotating the legs. The vastus lateralis, vastus medialis, and vastus intermedius work to extend the knees. Weakness in the medial hamstrings can cause the gluteus maximus to do more than its share of hip extension, in which case the legs externally rotate or abduct, or both.

Weakness in the pronators of the forearms or shortness in the supinators (or interosseus membrane) makes the elbows flare out to the sides and affects both the elbow and shoulder joints. The forearms should stay parallel to each other for the best alignment of action through the arms into the spine.

Breathing

Although the standard instruction is to inhale while entering into a back bend, it can be very helpful to enter into this basic back bend on an exhalation. For many people who are locked into a belly breathing pattern, their inhalation actually restricts thoracic extension and rib cage expansion (this is because a belly breath is accomplished by restricting rib movement while the diaphragm contracts).

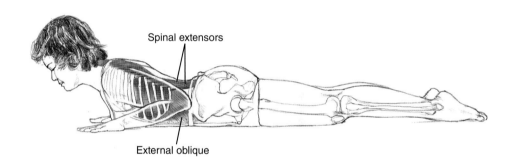

Spinal extensors

External oblique

Bhujangasana Variation

With Knees Flexed

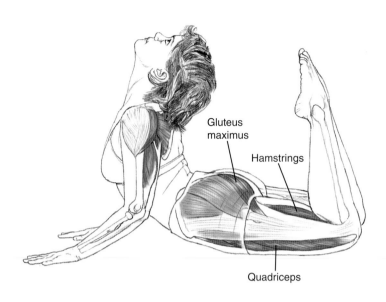

Gluteus maximus

Hamstrings

Quadriceps

Notes

In this position, the hamstrings are used for both actions of hip extension and knee flexion. This position of the legs puts the hamstrings at a very short working length, which greatly increases the chances of cramping in the muscles.

This position also makes it more likely that the outer fibers of the gluteus maximus will fire to help with the hip extension, which will also externally rotate and abduct the legs. Often, a student who can keep the legs adducted and parallel when the knees are extended will find it much more challenging when the knees are flexed. In this position, all of the quadriceps are lengthened, and the range of motion in the rectus femoris can restrict the range of motion in knee flexion too.

Dhanurasana

Bow Pose

don-your-AHS-anna

dhanu = bow

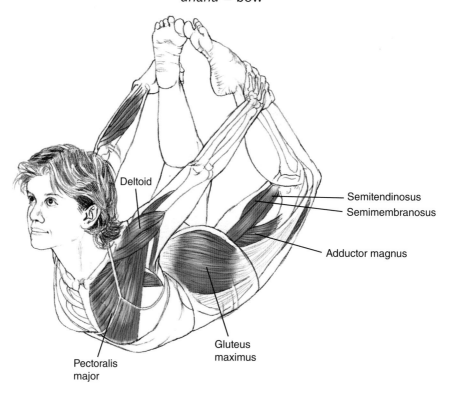

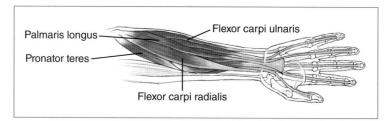

Classification

Symmetrical prone backward-bending pose

Skeletal joint actions		
Spine	**Upper limbs**	**Lower limbs**
Extension	Scapular adduction; shoulder internal rotation, extension, and adduction; elbow extension; forearm pronation; finger and hand flexion	SI joint counternutation, hip extension and adduction, knee flexion, ankle plantar flexion

Muscular joint actions

Spine

Concentric contraction	Eccentric contraction
To extend spine:	**To prevent overmobilization of lumbar spine:**
Spinal extensors	Psoas minor, abdominal muscles

Upper limbs

Concentric contraction		Eccentric contraction
To adduct scapula:	**To extend shoulder:**	**To resist pull of arm on scapula:**
Rhomboids	Posterior deltoid, teres	Pectoralis major and minor, coracobrachialis,
To stabilize shoulder joint:	major, triceps brachii	anterior deltoid
Rotator cuff	**To pronate forearm:**	
	Pronator quadratus and teres	

Lower limbs

Concentric contraction	
To extend, adduct, and internally rotate hip and flex knee:	**To plantar flex ankle:**
Hamstrings, adductor magnus, gluteus maximus	Soleus

Notes

The fronts of the shoulder joints are structurally vulnerable in this position. If the scapulae are not mobilized in the direction of adduction and some elevation, too much pressure could be put into the anterior shoulder joints, resulting in an overmobilization of the subscapularis or damage to the joint capsules. Because this is a bound pose, the pressure into these vulnerable joints is greater.

This pose can be explored in a variety of ways by emphasizing different actions: by deepening the action in the spine, by increasing hip extension, or by using knee extension to deepen spinal and hip extension. The balance of actions in the hips and knees will be affected depending on whether the hamstrings or the quadriceps are more activated. Because this is a bound pose, with the hands grasping the ankles, it is also possible to put too much pressure into the knees. Thus, the alignment of the legs at the hips and the activation of the feet are important to maintain the integrity of the knees.

Breathing

It is a common practice to rock back and forth in this pose by pushing the belly into the floor with each inhalation. It is also interesting to practice not rocking by directing the inhalation into the already expanded chest region.

Salabhasana

Locust Pose

sha-la-BAHS-anna

salabha = grasshopper, locust

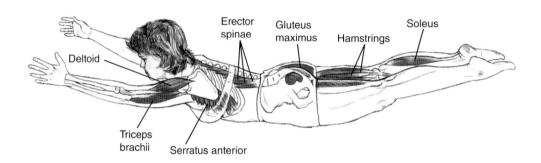

Classification

Symmetrical prone backward-bending pose

Skeletal joint actions		
Spine	**Upper limbs**	**Lower limbs**
Extension	Scapular upward rotation, elevation, and abduction; shoulder flexion; elbow extension	SI joint counternutation, hip extension and adduction, knee extension, ankle plantar flexion

Muscular joint actions

Spine

Concentric contraction

To extend spine:
Spinal extensors

Upper limbs

Concentric contraction

To upwardly rotate and elevate scapula:
Serratus anterior

To stabilize shoulder joint:
Rotator cuff

To flex shoulder:
Anterior deltoid, biceps brachii (long head)

To extend elbow:
Triceps brachii

To pronate forearm:
Pronator quadratus and teres

Lower limbs

Concentric contraction

To extend, adduct, and internally rotate hip:
Hamstrings, adductor magnus, gluteus
    maximus

To extend knee:
Vastii

To plantar flex ankle:
Soleus

Notes

It can be a challenge to lift the arms in this relationship to gravity, with the spine in exten-sion. If the latissimus dorsi are used to extend the spine (rather than the deeper, intrinsic spinal muscles), they will inhibit the movement in the arms.

This position of the legs uses a complex interaction among adductors, medial rotators, and hip extensors. This is because many of the muscle actions that lift and support the body in this position create other actions that must be neutralized by opposing or syner-gistic muscles. For example, because the gluteus maximus, a powerful hip extensor, also externally rotates the legs, it's preferable to use the hamstrings for hip extension. People will have different priorities, or challenges, depending on where they start and their preexisting patterns of strength and weakness as well as flexibility and tightness.

Breathing

To rock, or not to rock? All the weight of the body is brought to bear on the abdomen in this variation. While holding the pose for several breaths, the body rocks back and forth with the action of the diaphragm if the primary breathing pattern is belly breathing. An interesting challenge is to keep from rocking, which necessitates a release in the thoracic structures and diaphragm, allowing the floor to push into the abdomen, rather than the abdomen to push into the floor.

Viparita Salabhasana

Full Locust Pose

vip-par-ee-tah sha-la-BAHS-anna

viparita = reversed, inverted; *salabha* = grasshopper, locust

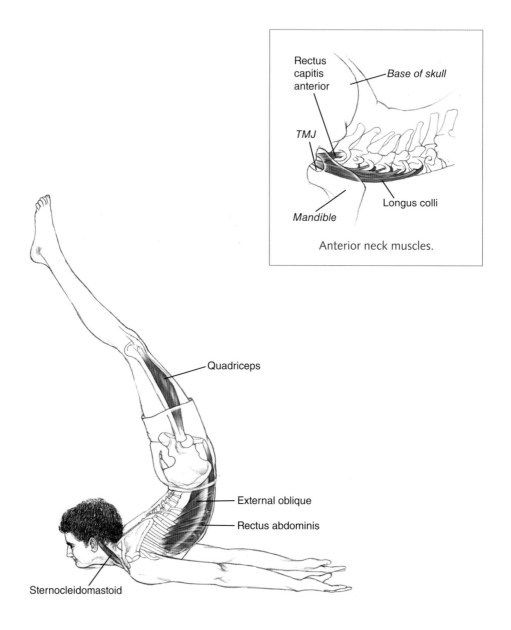

Rectus capitis anterior

Base of skull

TMJ

Longus colli

Mandible

Anterior neck muscles.

Quadriceps

External oblique

Rectus abdominis

Sternocleidomastoid

Classification

Symmetrical prone backward-bending pose

Skeletal joint actions		
Spine	**Upper limbs**	**Lower limbs**
Extension	Scapular downward rotation, elevation, and abduction; shoulder internal rotation, flexion, and adduction; elbow extension	SI joint counternutation, hip extension and adduction, knee extension, ankle plantar flexion

Muscular joint actions

Spine

Eccentric contraction

To keep pelvis and leg from dropping into floor:
Abdominal muscles, psoas minor

To prevent hypermobilizing of cervical spine:
Anterior neck muscles

Upper limbs

Concentric contraction

To stabilize shoulder joint:
Rotator cuff

To abduct scapula:
Serratus anterior

To flex shoulder and lift body weight:
Pectoralis major, anterior deltoid, biceps brachii, coracobrachialis

Lower limbs

Eccentric contraction

To keep leg from dropping behind head:
Psoas major, vastii

Notes

What it takes to move into this pose is almost completely the opposite of what it takes to remain in it. Lifting the weight of the body into spinal extension requires a strong, integrated action of the arms and spinal extensors. Once past vertical, gravity pulls the weight of the body into extension, so the trunk flexors must engage to prevent hyperextension. Based on their balance of strength and flexibility in the extensor and flexor muscle groups, some people may have the ability to get into full locust but not to sustain it, whereas others can't get there themselves but can stay there if assisted into the pose.

(continued)

Breathing

The standard instruction to inhale while entering into a back bend can be counterproductive here. This is because a strong contraction of the diaphragm draws the base of the rib cage and lumbar spine toward the central tendon. This can create considerable resistance to the lengthening in the deep front line of the body. Exhaling while lifting the body into the pose works better for many people.

Remaining in the pose requires the abdominal wall to be both lengthened and engaged, which can limit abdominal breath movement, while the actions that synergize the push of the arms into the floor tend to limit thoracic excursion. In addition, having the neck in weight-bearing extension can add resistance to the airway—not to mention that all of this is happening in an inverted position. All in all, this is a very challenging position to breathe in. Efficiency of effort is the key.

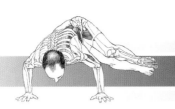

ARM SUPPORT POSES

In spite of their obvious similarities, the upper and lower extremities of the human body have evolved to perform different functions. The structures of the foot, knee, hip, and pelvis point to their functions of support and locomotion.

The highly mobile structures of the hand, elbow, and shoulder girdle have evolved to reach and grasp and are less ideally suited to weight bearing. In fact, when you compare the proportional structures of the hand and foot, you see an inverse relationship between the weight-bearing and articular structures within them.

In the foot, the heavy, dense tarsal bones comprise half the length of its structure. Adding to this the weight-bearing function of the metatarsals, it can be said that four fifths of the foot's structure is dedicated to weight bearing. The foot's phalangeal structures (the toes) contribute only one fifth of its total length.

These proportions are completely reversed in the hand, where half the length of the structure is composed of the highly mobile phalangeal (finger) bones. The hand's metacarpals are also very mobile (compared to the metatarsals), whereas the relatively immobile carpals (wrist bones) comprise only one fifth of the total length of the hand. This means that even if you effectively recruit the metacarpals in arm support, you still have only half the length of the hand structured for weight bearing.

When you use the upper limbs in weight-bearing poses, you have to take into account the fact that they are at a structural disadvantage and take extra care in preparation and execution.

On the other hand, taking the time to learn how to organize support through the hands and upper limbs can be a wonderful recuperation for the ways in which people stress their hands, arms, shoulders, and upper backs while sitting at desks and using computers.

Adho Mukha Svanasana

Downward-Facing Dog Pose

AH-doh MOO-kah shvah-NAHS-anna

adho = downward; *mukha* = face; *shvana* = dog

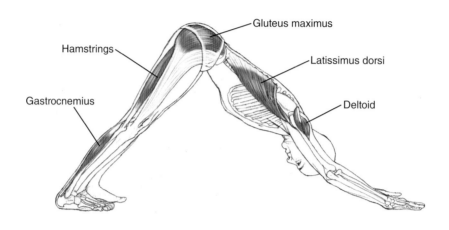

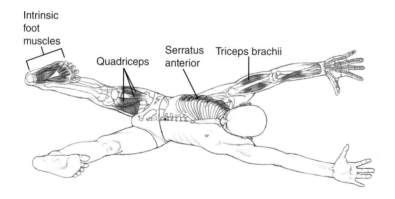

Classification

Symmetrical inverted arm support pose

Skeletal joint actions		
Spine	**Upper limbs**	**Lower limbs**
Neutral spine	Scapular upward rotation and elevation, shoulder flexion, elbow extension, forearm pronation, wrist dorsiflexion	SI joint nutation, hip flexion, knee extension, ankle dorsiflexion

Muscular joint actions

Spine

To calibrate concentric and eccentric contractions to maintain neutral alignment of spine:
Spinal extensors and flexors

Upper limbs

Concentric contraction

To upwardly rotate and abduct scapula on rib cage: Serratus anterior	**To extend elbow:** Triceps brachii
To stabilize shoulder joint: Rotator cuff	**To pronate forearm:** Pronator quadratus and teres
To flex shoulder: Deltoid, biceps brachii (long head)	**To maintain integrity of hand:** Intrinsic muscles of wrist and hand

Lower limbs

Concentric contraction	*Eccentric contraction*
To internally rotate, adduct, and move femur back in hip socket: Adductor magnus	**To prevent overarticulating in hip joint:** Hamstrings
To extend knee: Articularis genu, vastii	
To maintain arches of foot without inhibiting dorsiflexion of ankle: Intrinsic muscles of foot	

Notes

There are many approaches to working with this pose. Fundamentally, it is a great opportunity to observe the effects of the arms and legs on the spine.

Assuming the spine is in neutral extension or axial extension, then there is flexion in both the shoulder joints and the hip joints and extension in the elbows and knees.

The latissimus dorsi often try to help in the action of the arms, but these muscles depress and internally rotate the shoulders (the opposite of the desired action), which can create an impingement at the acromion process.

The pronators are active in the forearms, but if rotation between the radius and ulna is limited, this restriction can translate into overarticulation in the elbows or wrists, or internal rotation of the arms at the shoulder joints—all common sites of injury for practitioners of vinyasa styles of yoga that employ repetitive downward-facing dogs in sun salutations.

As in the foot and leg, the intrinsic action in the hand is essential for the integration of the whole arm. Essentially, each hand must act as much like a foot as possible by maintaining its arch.

Breathing

From the perspective of the breath, this pose is an inversion. Because inversions naturally move the diaphragm cranially, the exhaling action of the abdominal muscles can be quite deep. If the lower abdominal action is maintained when initiating the inhalation (mula bandha), the thoracic structures are encouraged to mobilize, which can be quite challenging in an arm support pose.

Urdhva Mukha Svanasana

Upward-Facing Dog Pose

OORD-vah MOO-kah shvah-NAHS-anna

urdhva = rising or tending upward, raised, elevated; *mukha* = face; *shvana* = dog

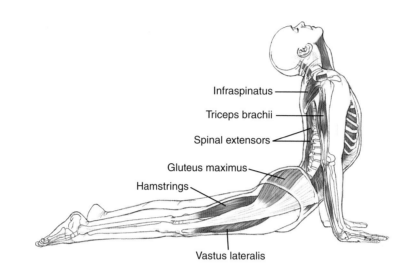

Infraspinatus

Triceps brachii

Spinal extensors

Gluteus maximus

Hamstrings

Vastus lateralis

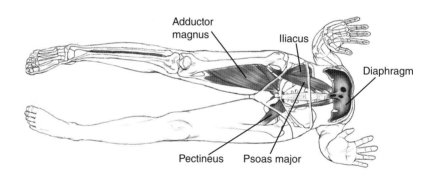

Adductor magnus

Iliacus

Diaphragm

Pectineus   Psoas major

Classification

Symmetrical backward-bending arm support pose

Skeletal joint actions		
Spine	**Upper limbs**	**Lower limbs**
Extension	Shoulder extension and adduction, elbow extension, forearm pronation	SI joint counternutation, hip extension and adduction, knee extension, ankle plantar flexion

226

Muscular joint actions

Spine

Concentric contraction	Eccentric contraction
To extend spine, especially thoracic curve: Spinal extensors	**To prevent overmobilization of lumbar spine:** Psoas minor, abdominal muscles
	To resist hyperextension in cervical spine as head extends: Anterior neck muscles

Upper limbs

Concentric contraction

To stabilize scapula on rib cage and translate push of arm into clavicle: Serratus anterior	**To extend shoulder:** Posterior deltoid
To stabilize shoulder joint: Rotator cuff	**To extend shoulder and elbow:** Triceps brachii
	To pronate forearm: Pronator quadratus and teres

Lower limbs

Concentric contraction

To extend, adduct, and internally rotate hip: Hamstrings, adductor magnus	**To plantar flex ankle:** Soleus
To extend knee: Articularis genu, vastii	

Notes

If the goal is to have extension distributed throughout the whole spine, there will need to be more action in the thoracic region and less in the lumbar and cervical regions. This translates into concentric work for the extensors in the thoracic spine and eccentric work for the flexors in the cervical and lumbar spines.

The latissimus dorsi are not so helpful in this pose, because they can fix the scapulae on the rib cage and inhibit extension in the thoracic spine. They also produce internal rotation of the humerus and downward rotation of the scapulae, which oppose the actions of this pose.

Depending on where restrictions are, the humerus can be drawn into either internal or external rotation.

The pronators in the forearms and the intrinsic muscles of each hand distribute pressure through the whole hand to protect the heel of each hand and decrease pressure in each wrist.

Breathing

As the counterpose to adho mukha svanasana (page 224), which is often done while exhaling, this pose is related to the expansive action of inhaling. Holding this pose for several breaths allows the inhaling action to deepen the extension in the thoracic spine, whereas the exhaling action can assist in stabilizing the lumbar and cervical curves.

Adho Mukha Vrksasana

Downward-Facing Tree Pose

AH-doh MOO-kah vrik-SHAHS-anna

adho = downward; *mukha* = face; *vrksa* = tree

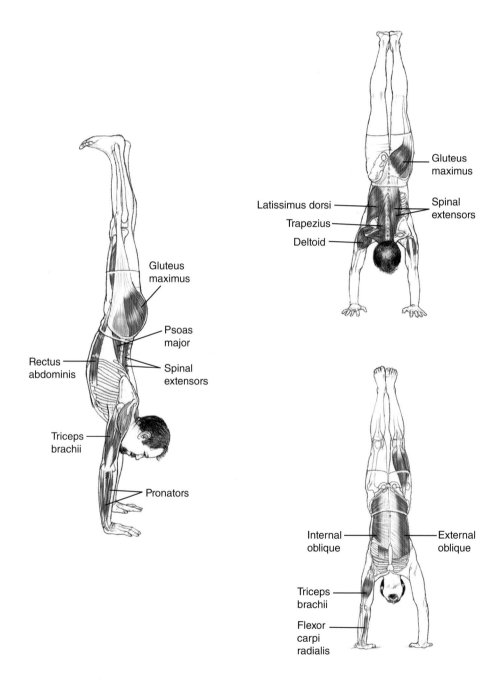

Gluteus maximus

Latissimus dorsi

Trapezius

Deltoid

Spinal extensors

Gluteus maximus

Psoas major

Rectus abdominis

Spinal extensors

Triceps brachii

Pronators

Internal oblique

External oblique

Triceps brachii

Flexor carpi radialis

Classification

Symmetrical inverted balancing arm support pose

Skeletal joint actions

Spine	Upper limbs	Lower limbs
Cervical extension, slight thoracic and lumbar extension	Scapular upward rotation and abduction, shoulder flexion, elbow extension, forearm pronation, wrist dorsiflexion	Hip neutral extension and adduction, knee extension, ankle dorsiflexion

Muscular joint actions

Spine

To calibrate concentric and eccentric contractions to maintain neutral alignment of spine:
Spinal extensors and flexors

Upper limbs

Concentric contraction

To upwardly rotate and abduct scapula on rib cage: Serratus anterior **To stabilize shoulder joint:** Rotator cuff **To flex shoulder:** Deltoid, biceps brachii (long head)	**To extend elbow:** Triceps brachii **To pronate forearm:** Pronator quadratus and teres **To maintain integrity of hand:** Intrinsic muscles of wrist and hand

Lower limbs

Concentric contraction	*Eccentric contraction*
To extend, adduct, and internally rotate leg to neutral: Hamstrings, adductor magnus, gluteus maximus	**To resist leg falling back:** Psoas major, iliacus

Notes

If the latissimus dorsi are tight, the flexion and upward rotation of the scapulae are inhibited, and the lumbar spine might hyperextend instead.

It's very challenging to maintain the integrity of the hands with all the weight of the body balancing on them, but it's essential in this pose because collapsing into the wrist or heel of the hand is quite dangerous for the carpal tunnel and the nerves passing through it.

For hypermobile students, it is especially important to find the strength of deep, intrinsic muscles so that the pose doesn't become rigid, but is both stable and fluid—in other words, it is available for breathing.

Breathing

This can be one of the most difficult poses in which to breathe effectively because of the challenges of balancing, inverting, and doing strong upper-body actions. Many people instinctively hold the breath, partly out of fear, but also because of a need to stabilize the movements of the spine. Of course, to maintain this balance for more than a few seconds, the breath must be integrated into the pose—not necessarily as deep, full breaths, but as efficient breaths that don't disrupt the balancing or stabilizing actions of the core musculature.

Chaturanga Dandasana

Four-Limbed Stick Pose

chaht-tour-ANG-ah dan-DAHS-anna

chatur = four; *anga* = limb; *danda* = staff, stick

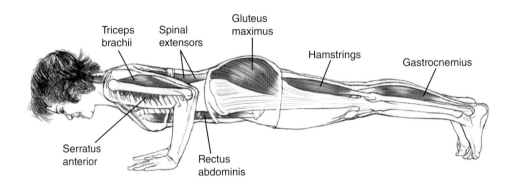

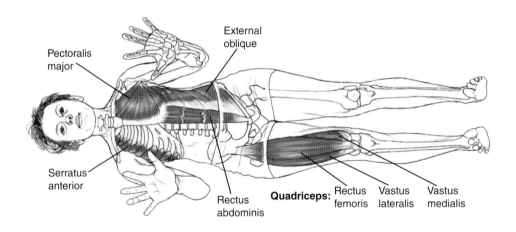

Classification

Symmetrical arm support pose

Skeletal joint actions		
Spine	**Upper limbs**	**Lower limbs**
Neutral spine	Scapular abduction, elbow flexion, forearm pronation, wrist dorsiflexion	Hip neutral extension and adduction, knee extension, ankle dorsiflexion

Muscular joint actions

Spine

To calibrate concentric and eccentric contractions to maintain neutral alignment of spine:
Spinal extensors and flexors

Upper limbs

Concentric contraction	*Eccentric contraction*
To prevent scapular winging: Serratus anterior **To stabilize and protect shoulder joint:** Rotator cuff, deltoid **To pronate forearm:** Pronator quadratus and teres **To maintain integrity of hand:** Intrinsic muscles of wrist and hand	**To resist extension of shoulder created by pull of gravity:** Pectoralis major and minor, coracobrachialis **To extend elbow:** Triceps brachii

Lower limbs

Concentric contraction	
To maintain neutral hip extension and adduction: Hamstrings, adductor magnus, gluteus maximus **To adduct hip:** Gracilis	**To extend knee:** Articularis genu, vastii **To create dorsiflexion:** Tibialis anterior **To support weight of leg on toes:** Intrinsic and extrinsic foot muscles

Notes

Weakness in the pose can appear in the lower body as lumbar hyperextension combined with hip flexion. To counter this, the hip extension action of the hamstrings is important.

In the upper body, weakness in the triceps brachii and serratus anterior can show up as a downward rotation of the scapulae and an overuse of the pectoralis major and minor.

Depressing the scapulae by recruiting the latissimus dorsi can give a feeling of strength in the back, but it contributes to hyperextension of the lumbar spine and a downward rotation of the scapulae.

Breathing

Maintaining this position relative to gravity calls into play virtually all the respiratory muscles, along with the arms and shoulder girdle. This degree of muscular effort produces a strong stabilizing effect on the movements of the diaphragm, which operate against considerable resistance. Progress in this pose consists of making the muscular effort as efficient as possible, which results in the ability to maintain both the alignment and smooth breathing for increasingly longer periods of time.

Bakasana

Crow Pose, Crane Pose

bak-AHS-anna

baka = crow, crane, heron

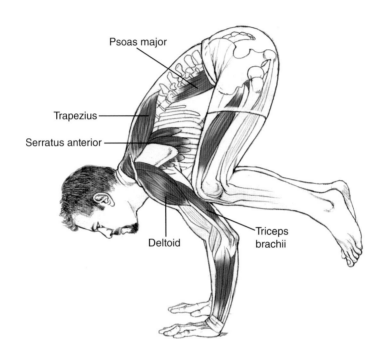

Psoas major

Trapezius

Serratus anterior

Deltoid

Triceps
brachii

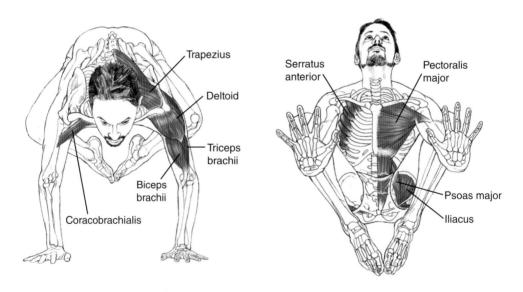

Trapezius

Deltoid

Triceps
brachii

Biceps
brachii

Coracobrachialis

Serratus
anterior

Pectoralis
major

Psoas major

Iliacus

Classification

Symmetrical balancing arm support pose

Skeletal joint actions

Spine	Upper limbs	Lower limbs
Cervical extension, thoracic and lumbar flexion	Scapular abduction, shoulder flexion and adduction, elbow flexion moving toward extension, forearm pronation, wrist dorsiflexion	SI joint nutation, hip flexion and adduction, knee flexion

Muscular joint actions

Spine

Concentric contraction

To extend cervical spine:
Rectus capitis posterior, obliquus capitis superior

To create deep flexion in lumbar spine:
Psoas major (upper fibers), psoas minor, abdominal muscles, pelvic floor

Upper limbs

Concentric contraction

To abduct scapula:
Serratus anterior, pectoralis major and minor, coracobrachialis

To stabilize and protect shoulder joint:
Rotator cuff, deltoid

To extend elbow:
Triceps brachii

To pronate forearm:
Pronator quadratus and teres

To maintain integrity of hand:
Intrinsic muscles of wrist and hand

Lower limbs

Concentric contraction

To flex hip:
Psoas major, iliacus

To adduct and flex hip:
Pectineus, adductor longus and brevis

To flex knee:
Lower hamstrings

Notes

In bird poses (crow, eagle, rooster, peacock, etc.), common factors are flexion of the thoracic spine, abduction of the scapulae, and extension of the cervical spine. These actions require precision and strength in the muscles of the spine to achieve cervical extension without engaging the trapezius, which interferes with the action of the scapulae and arms.

Although the knees initially widen to come into this position, the final action of the legs is adduction, to hug the knees to the sides of the upper arms or outer shoulders.

Breathing

Because the thoracic region is maintained in flexion, breath movements in the rib cage are minimized in this pose. The lower abdomen is also stabilized somewhat by the deep abdominal and hip flexor action, but the upper abdomen is relatively free to move.

Parsva Bakasana

Side Crow Pose, Side Crane Pose

parsh-vah bak-AHS-anna

parsva = side; *baka* = crow, crane, heron

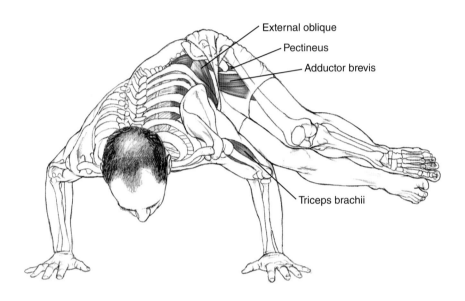

External oblique

Pectineus

Adductor brevis

Triceps brachii

Classification

Asymmetrical twisting balancing arm support pose

Skeletal joint actions		
Spine	**Upper limbs**	**Lower limbs**
Cervical extension, rotation	Scapular abduction, shoulder flexion and adduction, elbow flexion moving toward extension, forearm pronation, wrist dorsiflexion	Hip flexion and adduction, knee flexion

Muscular joint actions

Spine

Concentric contraction

To extend cervical spine:
Rectus capitis posterior, obliquus capitis superior

To rotate spine:
Internal oblique, erector spinae (bottom side); external oblique, multifidi, rotatores (top side)

Upper limbs

Concentric contraction

To abduct scapula:
Serratus anterior, pectoralis major and minor, coracobrachialis

To stabilize and protect shoulder joint:
Rotator cuff, deltoid

To extend elbow:
Triceps brachii

To pronate forearm:
Pronator quadratus and teres

To maintain integrity of hand:
Intrinsic muscles of wrist and hand

Lower limbs

Concentric contraction

To flex hip:
Psoas major, iliacus

To adduct and flex hip:
Pectineus, adductor longus and brevis

Notes

In this rotated pose the spine is more extended than in bakasana (page 232). If the knees separate in this pose, the rotation is happening more in the hip joints than in the spine.

Breathing

Breathing in this pose is similar to that in bakasana, but even more restricted because of the twisting of the spine.

Astavakrasana

Eight-Angle Pose

AHSH-tak-vah-KRAHS-anna

ashta = eight; *vakra* = crooked, curved, bent

Astavakra was a very learned sage whose mother attended Vedic chanting classes while pregnant. While he was in his mother's womb, he winced at eight of his father's mispronunciations of Vedic prayers, and was thus born with eight bends in his body.

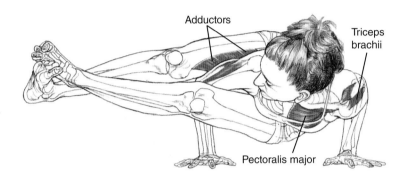

Classification

Asymmetrical twisting arm support pose

Skeletal joint actions		
Spine	**Upper limbs**	**Lower limbs**
Cervical extension, rotation	Scapular abduction, shoulder flexion and adduction, elbow flexion moving toward extension, forearm pronation, wrist dorsiflexion	Hip flexion and adduction, knee extension, ankle dorsiflexion, foot eversion

Muscular joint actions

Spine

Concentric contraction

To extend cervical spine:
Rectus capitis posterior, obliquus capitis superior

To rotate spine:
Internal oblique, erector spinae (bottom side); external oblique, multifidi, rotatores (top side)

Upper limbs

Concentric contraction

To abduct scapula:
Serratus anterior, pectoralis major and minor, coracobrachialis

To stabilize and protect shoulder joint:
Rotator cuff, deltoid

To extend elbow:
Triceps brachii

To pronate forearm:
Pronator quadratus and teres

To maintain integrity of hand:
Intrinsic muscles of wrist and hand

Lower limbs

Concentric contraction

To flex hip:
Psoas major, iliacus

To adduct and flex hip:
Pectineus, adductor longus and brevis

To extend knee:
Articularis genu, vastii

To dorsiflex ankle:
Tibialis anterior

To evert foot:
Peroneals

Notes

This pose requires the same action in the spine as parsva bakasana (page 234), although the spine is often slightly more extended (toward neutral) in astavakrasana, which allows for a more even distribution of the rotation through the spine.

In astavakrasana, the binding of the feet keeps the legs symmetrical. This symmetry in the legs and hip joints means that the rotation has to happen more in the spine and less in the hip joints. With the wrapping of the legs around the arm, less twist is needed than in parsva bakasana, because the bottom leg doesn't have to move to the top of the arm, but stays underneath it.

As in ardha matsyendrasana (page 150), if the spine does not rotate, potentially risky compensatory twisting can occur through overmobilizing the scapulae on the rib cage.

Also, the wrapping of the legs around the arm creates a fairly stable pivot point. The challenge of this pose (if one can do parsva bakasana) is more about balance and flexibility than strength. The extended legs in this pose might make the counterbalance on the support of the arms challenging.

Breathing

As compared to parsva bakasana, in which the body weight is lifted and supported on the upper arms, astavakrasana requires you to suspend the weight of the lower body from the support of the upper arms. It's interesting to examine which pose affords easier breathing. Which pose requires more or less expenditure of energy, and which offers more freedom of movement for the diaphragm?

Mayurasana
Peacock Pose

ma-your-AHS-anna

mayura = peacock

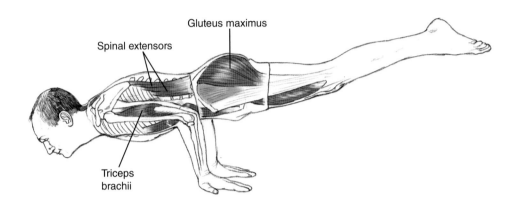

Classification

Symmetrical arm support pose

Skeletal joint actions		
Spine	**Upper limbs**	**Lower limbs**
Cervical extension, thoracic flexion, lumbar extension	Scapular abduction, shoulder adduction, elbow flexion, forearm supination, wrist dorsiflexion	Hip extension and adduction, knee extension, ankle plantar flexion

Muscular joint actions

Spine

Concentric contraction

To extend cervical spine:
Rectus capitis posterior, obliquus capitis superior

To flex lower thoracic spine:
Psoas major (upper fibers)

To extend lumbar spine:
Spinal extensors (lower fibers)

Upper limbs

Concentric contraction	*Eccentric contraction*
To abduct scapula: Serratus anterior, pectoralis major and minor, coracobrachialis	**To stabilize elbow:** Triceps brachii
To stabilize and protect shoulder joint: Rotator cuff, deltoid	
To stabilize elbow: Biceps brachii, brachialis	
To supinate forearm: Supinator	
To maintain integrity of hand: Intrinsic muscles of wrist and hand	

Lower limbs

Concentric contraction	
To extend, adduct, and internally rotate hip: Hamstrings, adductor magnus, gluteus maximus	**To extend knee:** Articularis genu, vastii **To plantar flex ankle:** Soleus

Notes

As in other bird poses (eagle, crow, rooster, etc.), mayurasana involves flexion of the thoracic spine, abduction of the scapulae, and extension of the cervical spine. It's unusual to balance on the arms with the forearms supinated. This changes the action in the elbows, and brings the biceps brachii much more into use.

A variation of mayurasana with the legs in padmasana (lotus) is generally easier to do because the lever of the legs is shortened by folding them in.

Breathing

The pressure of the elbows into the abdomen stimulates the organs. Many benefits have traditionally been ascribed to this effect. All the abdominal muscles activate to resist the pressure of the elbows into the viscera. The abdominal organs are being strongly squeezed from front and back, as well as from above and below, by the respiratory and pelvic diaphragms.

Considering how much muscular energy is expended to maintain this pose and the minimal amount of breathing it permits, it's no wonder that it is rarely held for more than a few breaths. The lungs in their limited capacity are simply unable to supply enough oxygen for that degree of muscular effort.

Pincha Mayurasana

Feathered Peacock Pose

pin-cha ma-your-AHS-anna

pincha = a feather of a tail; *mayura* = peacock

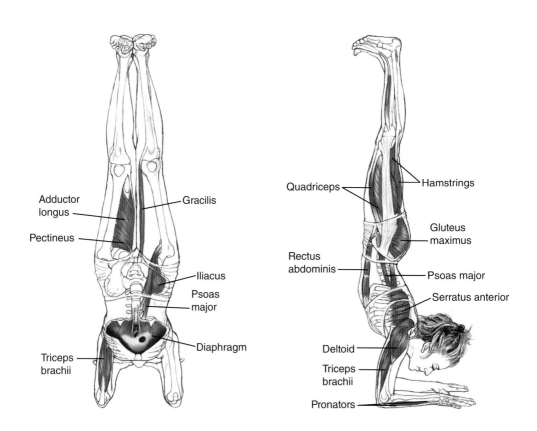

Adductor longus

Gracilis

Pectineus

Iliacus

Psoas major

Diaphragm

Triceps brachii

Quadriceps

Hamstrings

Gluteus maximus

Rectus abdominis

Psoas major

Serratus anterior

Deltoid

Triceps brachii

Pronators

Classification

Symmetrical inverted balancing arm support pose

Skeletal joint actions

Spine	Upper limbs	Lower limbs
Extension	Scapular upward rotation, elevation, and abduction; shoulder flexion and adduction; elbow flexion; forearm pronation	Hip adduction and neutral extension, knee extension, ankle dorsiflexion

Muscular joint actions

Spine

Concentric contraction	Eccentric contraction
To lift head away from floor: Rectus capitis posterior, obliquus capitis superior **To maintain extension of spine and keep from falling into flexion:** Spinal extensors	**To keep from falling into extension:** Psoas major (upper fibers), psoas minor, abdominal muscles

Upper limbs

Concentric contraction	Eccentric contraction
To upwardly rotate, abduct, and elevate scapula: Serratus anterior **To stabilize and protect shoulder joint:** Rotator cuff, deltoid **To resist shoulder extension:** Anterior deltoid **To flex and adduct shoulder:** Biceps brachii, anterior deltoid **To pronate forearm:** Pronator quadratus and teres **To maintain integrity of hand:** Intrinsic muscles of wrist and hand	**To resist elbow flexion and falling onto face:** Triceps brachii

Lower limbs

Concentric contraction	Eccentric contraction
To maintain neutral hip extension and adduction: Hamstrings, adductor magnus, gluteus maximus **To adduct hip:** Gracilis **To extend knee:** Articularis genu, vastii **To create dorsiflexion:** Tibialis anterior	**To prevent leg falling backward:** Psoas major

(continued)

Notes

With stability in the shoulder joints themselves (through the engagement of the rotator cuffs), the scapulae are free to mobilize on the rib cage, and there can be more freedom in the thoracic spine to extend and in the rib cage to breathe. Mobility in the thoracic spine is important; much like in urdhva mukha svanasana (page 226), the more extension available in the thoracic spine, the less the lower back and cervical spine have to do.

If tightness in the forearms (either in the supinators or in the interosseus membranes between the radius and the ulna) restricts full pronation, the elbows swing open or the hands come together. This common forearm issue is often interpreted as tightness in the shoulders or weakness in the wrists.

Shortness in the latissimus dorsi can also pull the elbows wide by internally rotating the humerus. This can feel like tight shoulders, but can actually be addressed by side bending and other actions that lengthen the latissimus dorsi. Shortness in these muscles also causes too much lumbar extension and interferes with breathing.

Breathing

The base of support for this pose is formed by the forearms, rib cage, and thoracic spine, and these structures need to be quite stable to maintain balance. Because of this, excessive chest breathing might interfere with supporting a forearm stand. On the other hand, the weight of the legs and pelvis and the curve of the lumbar spine need to be stabilized by the abdominal muscles, making too much abdominal movement counterproductive. Because of these factors, a breathing pattern that moves equally and smoothly throughout the body is needed.

Salamba Sirsasana

Supported Headstand

sah-LOM-bah shear-SHAHS-anna

sa = with; *alamba* = that on which one rests or leans, support; *sirsa* = head

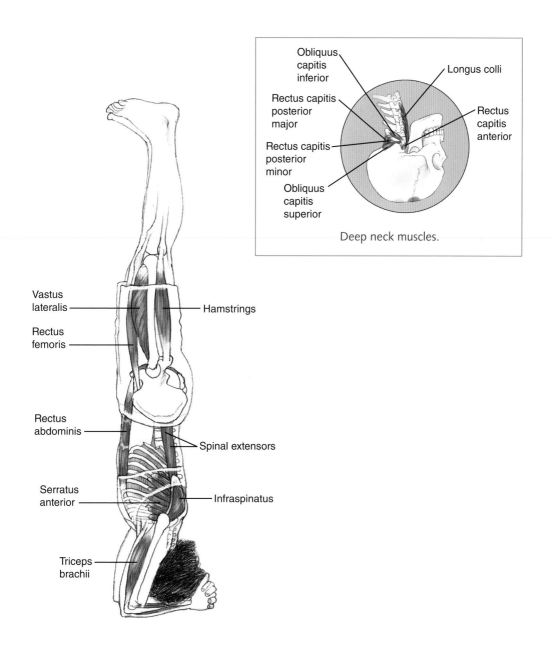

Obliquus capitis inferior

Longus colli

Rectus capitis posterior major

Rectus capitis anterior

Rectus capitis posterior minor

Obliquus capitis superior

Deep neck muscles.

Vastus lateralis

Hamstrings

Rectus femoris

Rectus abdominis

Spinal extensors

Serratus anterior

Infraspinatus

Triceps brachii

Classification

Symmetrical inverted balancing arm support pose

(continued)

Skeletal joint actions

Spine	Upper limbs	Lower limbs
Neutral spine	Scapular upward rotation; shoulder flexion and adduction; elbow flexion; neutral forearm, hand, and finger flexion	Hip adduction and neutral extension, knee extension, ankle dorsiflexion

Muscular joint actions

Spine

To calibrate concentric and eccentric contractions to maintain neutral alignment of spine:	To balance and stabilize atlanto-axial and atlanto-occipital joint:
Spinal extensors and flexors	Rectus capitis anterior, rectus capitis posterior major and minor, obliquus capitis superior and inferior, longus capitis and colli

Upper limbs

Concentric contraction	*Eccentric contraction*
To upwardly rotate scapula:	**To resist elbow flexion:**
Serratus anterior	Triceps brachii
To stabilize and protect shoulder joint:	
Rotator cuff, deltoid	
To maintain integrity of hand:	
Intrinsic muscles of wrist and hand	

Lower limbs

Concentric contraction	*Eccentric contraction*
To maintain neutral hip extension and adduction:	**To prevent leg falling backward:**
Hamstrings, adductor magnus, gluteus maximus	Psoas major
To adduct hip:	
Gracilis	
To extend knee:	
Articularis genu, vastii	
To create dorsiflexion:	
Tibialis anterior	

Notes

For some, the ideal placement of the weight on the skull is on the bregma—the juncture between the coronal and sagittal sutures, where the frontal bone meets the two parietal bones. This leads to a slightly more arched final position. Placing the weight more toward the crown of the head leads to a more neutral spine and more balanced action between the front and back of the body.

Many people have asymmetries and slight rotations in their spines, which become more apparent in this pose. Note the rotational shifts and other asymmetries in the illustration of the author in salamba sirsasana below.

It can be a challenge to find full hip extension in this pose. If the abdominal muscles are not strong enough, the hips can flex to keep the work of the pose in the back muscles instead of in the front.

Note: Contrary to popular notions of increased blood or oxygen flow to the brain in inversions, it should be noted that the body has very robust mechanisms that control the amount of blood delivered to any given region, irrespective of the orientation to gravity.

Regional changes in blood pressure have been observed based on inversion or compression of major blood vessels by body position, but this is a distinct issue from movement of blood volume and thus oxygen delivery.

That said, inversions do offer a very beneficial opportunity for increased venous return from the lower body, as well as improved lymph drainage—not to mention the benefits derived from inverting the action of the diaphragm.

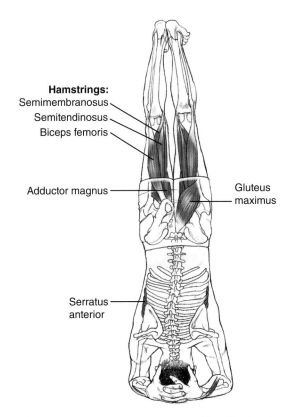

The author's asymmetries are exaggerated in salamba sirsasana.

(continued)

Even if you favor the bregma version of this pose and enter into the pose with straight legs with the intention to end up in a more arched position, the strength and coordination required to maintain salamba sirsasana safely demands certain skills that can be best developed by practicing the bent-leg entry into the pose. The key test is whether you can raise the weight off the feet without jumping and maintain the difficult pose known as acunchanasana (bent-legged headstand) for several breaths.

Breathing

When the support for salamba sirsasana is derived from the deeper intrinsic muscles of the spine, as well as the coordinated actions of the hamstrings, vastii, psoas minor, internal obliques, transversus abdominis, and serratus anterior, the

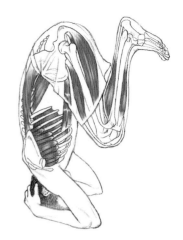

Acunchanasana.

weight forces of the body are more neutralized in gravity. Then, the muscular effort of remaining in the pose is minimized, and the breath is calm and efficient. At that point, the inverted nature of the diaphragm's action is emphasized because of the strong actions of the abdominal muscles and pelvic diaphragm, which help to stabilize the center of gravity over the base of support. All the internal organs, which anchor to the central tendon of the diaphragm, can move differently in inversions.

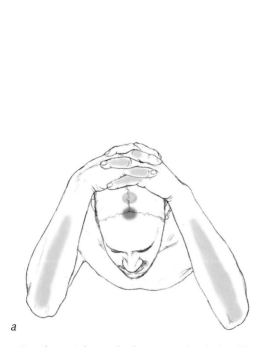

a

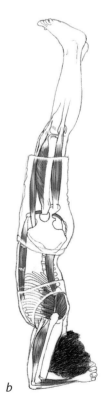

b

Supporting the weight on the bregma—the darker blue spot in figure *a*—results in the slightly more arched position in figure *b*. Supporting weight near the crown—the lighter blue spot in figure *a*—leads to a more neutral spine position.

Vrschikasana

Scorpion Pose

vrs-chee-KAHS-anna

vrschana = scorpion

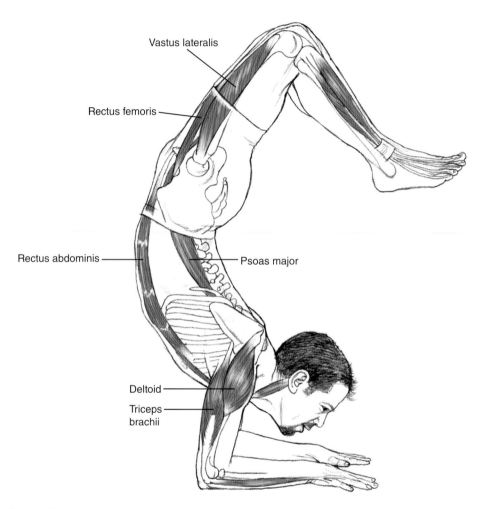

Vastus lateralis

Rectus femoris

Rectus abdominis

Psoas major

Deltoid

Triceps
brachii

Classification

Symmetrical inverted backward-bending arm support pose

Skeletal joint actions		
Spine	**Upper limbs**	**Lower limbs**
Extension	Scapular upward rotation, elevation, and adduction; shoulder flexion and adduction; elbow flexion; forearm pronation	Hip extension and adduction, knee flexion, ankle plantar flexion

(continued)

Muscular joint actions

Spine

Concentric contraction	Eccentric contraction
To lift head away from floor:	**To keep from falling into extension:**
Rectus capitis posterior, obliquus capitis superior	Psoas major (upper fibers), psoas minor, abdominal muscles
To maximize extension of spine:	
Spinal extensors	

Upper limbs

Concentric contraction	Eccentric contraction
To stabilize and protect shoulder joint:	**To stabilize scapula as it adducts:**
Rotator cuff, deltoid	Serratus anterior
To resist shoulder extension and adduct shoulder:	**To resist elbow flexion and falling onto face:**
Biceps brachii, anterior deltoid	Triceps brachii
To pronate forearm:	
Pronator quadratus and teres	
To maintain integrity of hand:	
Intrinsic muscles of wrist and hand	

Lower limbs

Concentric contraction	
To extend, adduct, and internally rotate hip and flex knee:	**To adduct hip and flex knee:**
Hamstrings, adductor magnus, gluteus maximus	Gracilis

Notes

Even though pincha mayurasana (page 240) is considered preparation for vrschikasana, vrschikasana can be an easier pose to balance in because of its lower center of gravity.

To deepen from pincha mayurasana into vrschikasana, the scapulae need to slide together on the back, which lowers the rib cage toward the floor and creates more mobility in the thoracic spine. The head can then lift and the thoracic spine can extend further. This also changes the pivot point for balancing from between the shoulders to closer toward the sacrum in the spine. The lifting of the head is important to shifting the balance point; otherwise, the legs might overbalance the pose backward, causing you to fall into a back bend.

As the knees bend and the feet move toward the head, the hamstrings are at their shortest working length. For this reason, they often cramp while trying to do this action.

As important as getting into this pose is the ability to get out of it and find the relative neutrality of pincha mayurasana again. It's a good idea to practice it in a manageable range, entering and exiting the pose with control.

Urdhva Dhanurasana

Upward Bow Pose, Wheel Pose

OORD-vah don-your-AHS-anna

urdhva = upward; *dhanu* = bow

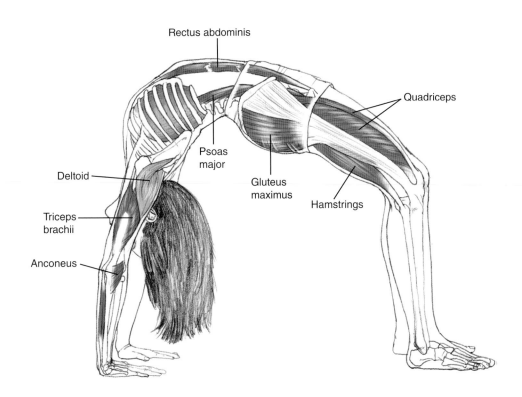

Classification

Symmetrical backward-bending arm support pose

(continued)

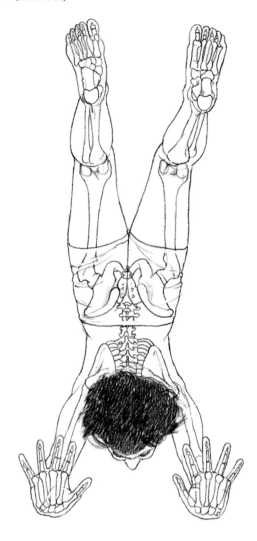

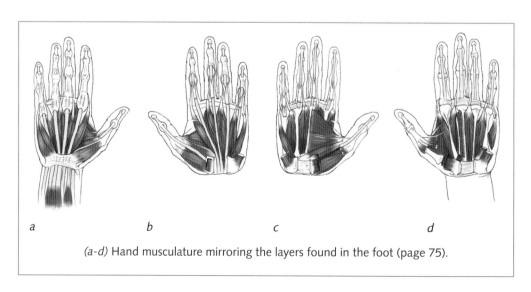

a   *b*   *c*   *d*

(a-d) Hand musculature mirroring the layers found in the foot (page 75).

Skeletal joint actions

Spine	Upper limbs	Lower limbs
Extension	Scapular upward rotation and elevation, shoulder flexion, elbow extension, forearm pronation, wrist dorsiflexion, hand and finger extension	Hip extension and adduction, knee flexion, ankle plantar flexion

Muscular joint actions

Spine

Concentric contraction	Eccentric contraction
To lift head away from floor:	**To keep from hyperextending lumbar spine:**
Rectus capitis posterior, obliquus capitis superior	Psoas minor, abdominals
To maximize extension of spine:	
Spinal extensors	

Upper limbs

Concentric contraction	
To upwardly rotate and elevate scapula:	**To extend elbow:**
Serratus anterior	Triceps brachii
To stabilize and protect shoulder joint:	**To pronate forearm:**
Rotator cuff, deltoid	Pronator quadratus and teres
To flex shoulder:	**To maintain integrity of hand:**
Biceps brachii, anterior deltoid	Intrinsic muscles of wrist and hand

Lower limbs

Concentric contraction	
To extend hip:	**To extend knee:**
Hamstrings, gluteus maximus	Articularis genu, vastii
To extend, adduct, and internally rotate hip:	
Adductor magnus, gracilis	

(continued)

Notes

The correct leg action is useful for getting into urdhva dhanurasana. When people use the quadriceps to try to extend the knees, it can create a pushing action that thrusts weight toward the head and arms, making it even harder to raise the upper body off the floor. Initiating the lift of the pelvis with more attention to hip extension can pull the weight of the body over the legs and make less work for the upper limbs.

Of the adductor group, the adductor magnus is most useful for urdhva dhanurasana because it creates hip extension and internal rotation along with adduction—all actions that support the alignment of the pose. The gluteus maximus is less useful for hip extension in this position because it can create external rotation, which can lead to compression in the sacrum and low-back pain.

The arms need to move freely overhead, and a combination of mobilizing the scapulae and stabilizing the rotation in the shoulder joints with the rotator cuffs creates the necessary balance. If the latissimus dorsi are short or overactive, they restrict the ability of the scapulae to upwardly rotate. This can force excessive action into the spine or shoulder joints.

Similarly, if the hips don't extend with ease, too much movement can be forced into the lumbar spine.

Breathing

Many students have been frustrated by their inability to take deep, full breaths in urdhva dhanurasana. The reason for this is simple: In this shape, the body is stabilized in a maximal inhalation, and there is very little one can do to expand further if attempting to inhale deeply. Quiet, relaxed breathing is preferable. The more efficient the muscle action in the pose is, the less oxygen you'll need to fuel the effort.

Vasisthasana

Side Plank Pose, Sage Vasistha's Pose

vah-sish-TAHS-anna

vasistha = a sage; most excellent, best, richest

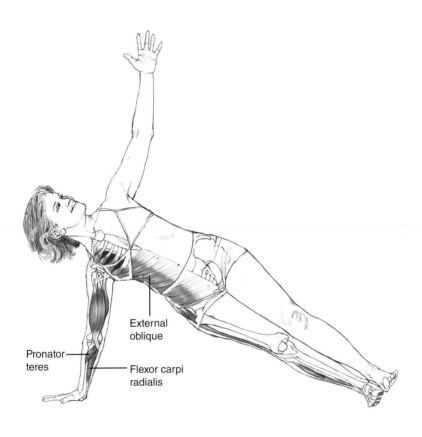

External oblique

Pronator teres

Flexor carpi radialis

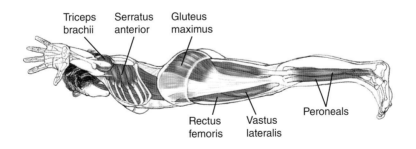

Triceps brachii

Serratus anterior

Gluteus maximus

Rectus femoris

Vastus lateralis

Peroneals

Classification

Asymmetrical balancing arm support pose

(continued)

Skeletal joint actions

Spine	Upper limbs			Lower limbs
		Bottom arm	**Top arm**	
Neutral spine	Neutral scapula, shoulder abduction, elbow extension	Forearm pronation, wrist dorsiflexion	Forearm and wrist neutral	Hip neutral extension and adduction, knee extension, ankle dorsiflexion

Muscular joint actions

Spine

Alternating concentric and eccentric contractions	Concentric contraction	Eccentric contraction
To maintain neutral alignment of spine: Spinal extensors and flexors	**To resist top hip twisting forward:** External oblique (top side); internal oblique (bottom side) **To turn head upward:** Splenius capitis (top side); sternocleidomastoid (bottom side) **To resist hip dropping to floor:** Quadratus lumborum (bottom side)	**To resist hip falling back:** Internal oblique (top side); external oblique (bottom side)

Upper limbs

Concentric contraction

To maintain scapula position on rib cage: Serratus anterior	**To extend elbow:** Triceps brachii
To stabilize and protect shoulder joint: Rotator cuff	**To pronate forearm:** Pronator quadratus and teres
To abduct shoulder: Deltoid	**To maintain integrity of hand:** Intrinsic muscles of wrist and hand

Lower limbs

Concentric contraction

To maintain neutral hip extension and adduction: Hamstrings, adductor magnus, gluteus maximus	**To create dorsiflexion:** Tibialis anterior
To extend knee: Articularis genu, vastii	**To evert foot:** Intrinsic and extrinsic foot muscles

Notes

The challenge of this pose is not one of flexibility, but instead how to maintain the neutral alignment of the spine and legs and the simple positions of the arms against the action of gravity. The asymmetrical relationship to gravity means that muscles have to work asymmetrically to create a symmetrical alignment of the body—essentially tadasana (page 72) turned on its side.

There are many ways that gravity pulls the body out of tadasana in this pose: The spine may twist, the hips may fall forward or the shoulders may fall back (or vice versa), the bottom scapula and bottom leg may both adduct, or the pelvis may fall to the floor. It's easy to overcompensate by lifting the hips too high or to create lateral flexion of the spine in either direction by either giving in to gravity or overresisting it.

Side plank pose is simple, but not easy.

Breathing

From the standpoint of the breath, this pose has much in common with niralamba sarvangasana (page 193). It is also a challenging balancing pose that requires a lot of stabilizing action in the abdominal and thoracic musculature. Side plank is a bit easier because the arms can be used for support and balance, but deep breathing might still have the effect of destabilizing the pose.

Efficiency—finding the minimum amount of effort necessary to maintain the position—allows the limited breath movements to supply just enough energy to sustain the pose.

Chatus Pada Pitham
Four-Footed Tabletop Pose

CHA-toos PA-da PEE-tham

chatur = four; *pada* = foot; *pitham* = stool, seat, chair, bench

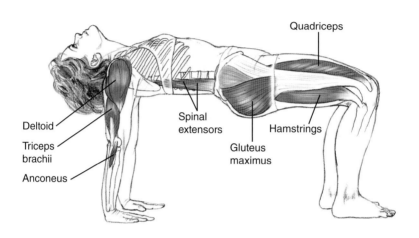

Quadriceps

Deltoid

Triceps
brachii

Anconeus

Spinal
extensors

Hamstrings

Gluteus
maximus

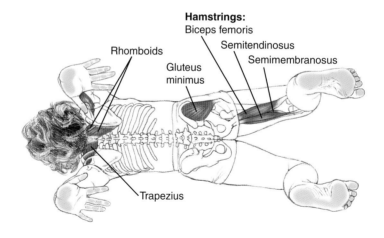

Hamstrings:
Biceps femoris

Semitendinosus

Semimembranosus

Rhomboids

Gluteus
minimus

Trapezius

Classification

Symmetrical arm support pose

Skeletal joint actions

Spine	Upper limbs	Lower limbs
Cervical extension, slight thoracic and lumbar extension	Scapular downward rotation, elevation, and adduction; shoulder extension; elbow extension; wrist dorsiflexion	SI joint counternutation, hip extension and adduction, knee flexion, ankle dorsiflexion

Muscular joint actions

Spine

Concentric contraction	Eccentric contraction
To extend spine, especially thoracic curve: Spinal extensors	**To resist hyperextension in cervical and lumbar spine:** Anterior neck muscles, psoas minor, abdominal muscles

Upper limbs

Concentric contraction	
To adduct, elevate, and downwardly rotate scapula: Rhomboids, levator scapulae	**To extend elbow:** Triceps brachii
To stabilize shoulder joint and prevent protraction of head of humerus: Rotator cuff	**To pronate forearm:** Pronator quadratus and teres
To extend and adduct shoulder joint: Triceps brachii (long head), teres major, posterior deltoid	**To maintain integrity of hand:** Intrinsic muscles of wrist and hand

Lower limbs

Concentric contraction	
To extend hip: Hamstrings, gluteus maximus	**To extend knee:** Articularis genu, vastii
To extend, adduct, and internally rotate hip: Adductor magnus, gracilis	

(continued)

Notes

Weakness in the hamstrings makes it difficult to create neutral extension of the hip joints, so many people use the quadriceps to extend the knees and push the feet into the floor. The problem here is that this tends to also create hip flexion, which obstructs the openings at the fronts of the hip joints. Overusing the gluteus maximus also externally rotates the hips, which the adductors counter, creating even more restriction at the hip joints.

Too much tightness in the pectoral region prevents the scapulae from moving into adduction and results in either too much movement in the shoulder joints or in flexion of the spine.

Breathing

Unlike urdhva dhanurasana (page 249), chatus pada pitham is not an extreme spinal extension that can restrict movement of the back of the thoracic cavity. However, the extension of the arms at the shoulder joints can restrict the movement of the front of the thoracic cavity, particularly if there is any tightness across the pectoral muscles. This might encourage the breath to move more into the abdomen. The combination of lifting action in the back body and release in the front body makes for an interesting opportunity to experiment by moving the breath around the abdominal and thoracic regions. Some breathing patterns have more of an effect on the stability of the pose, whereas others can assist in opening the upper rib cage.

Purvottanasana

Upward Plank Pose

POOR-vo-tan-AHS-anna

purva = front, east; *ut* = intense; *tan* = extend, stretch

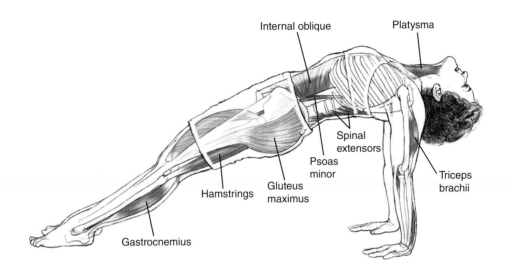

Classification

Symmetrical backward-bending arm support pose

Skeletal joint actions		
Spine	**Upper limbs**	**Lower limbs**
Extension	Scapular downward rotation, elevation, and adduction; shoulder extension; elbow extension; wrist dorsiflexion	SI joint counternutation, hip extension and adduction, knee extension, ankle plantar flexion

(continued)

Muscular joint actions	

Spine

Concentric contraction	*Eccentric contraction*
To extend spine, especially thoracic curve: Spinal extensors	**To resist hyperextension in cervical and lumbar spine:** Anterior neck muscles, psoas minor, abdominal muscles

Upper limbs

Concentric contraction	
To adduct, elevate, and downwardly rotate scapula: Rhomboids, levator scapulae **To stabilize shoulder joint and prevent protraction of head of humerus:** Rotator cuff **To extend and adduct shoulder joint:** Triceps brachii (long head), teres major, posterior deltoid	**To extend elbow:** Triceps brachii **To pronate forearm:** Pronator quadratus and teres **To maintain integrity of hand:** Intrinsic muscles of wrist and hand

Lower limbs

Concentric contraction	
To extend, adduct, and internally rotate hip: Hamstrings, adductor magnus, gluteus maximus	**To extend knee:** Articularis genu, vastii **To plantar flex ankle:** Soleus

Notes

Often in this pose there is too much lumbar extension and not enough hip extension, and the hip joints might even drop into flexion. The hamstrings should be the main extensors for the hip joints here, but if they are weak, the gluteus maximus can kick in. The problem with using the gluteus maximus is that it brings in external rotation, which is harder on the lower back.

If the hamstrings are too weak to do purvottanasana, then chatus pada pitham (page 256) is an excellent preparation.

The latissimus dorsi are not so helpful in this pose, because they can fix the scapulae on the rib cage and inhibit extension in the thoracic spine.

The actions needed in the scapulae, shoulder joints, and upper back are very similar to those in salamba sarvangasana (page 190), though in a different relationship to gravity and without the cervical flexion of the neck that brings the head forward.

Breathing

As in chatus pada pitham, the extension of the arms at the shoulder joints in purvottanasana can restrict the movement of the front of the thoracic cavity, particularly if there is any tightness across the pectoral muscles. This might encourage the breath to move more into the abdomen, which can be a challenge for the action needed to maintain hip and knee extension.

BIBLIOGRAPHY AND RESOURCES

BIBLIOGRAPHY

These are the references used for working on the poses:

Adler, S.S., D. Beckers, and M. Buck. 2003. *PNF in Practice.* 2nd ed. New York: Springer.

Clemente, C.D. 1997. *Anatomy: A Regional Atlas of the Human Body.* 4th ed. Philadelphia, PA: Lippincott Williams & Wilkins.

Gorman, David. 1995. *The Body Moveable.* 4th ed. Guelph, Ontario: Ampersand Press.

Kapit, W., and L.M. Elson. 1993. *The Anatomy Coloring Book.* 2nd ed. New York: HarperCollins College Publishers.

Kendall, F.P., E.K. McCreary, and P.G. Provance. 1993. *Muscles, Testing and Function.* 4th ed. Philadelphia, PA: Lippincott Williams & Wilkins.

Laban, R. 1966. *The Language of Movement: A Guidebook to Choreutics.* Great Britain: Macdonald and Evans.

Myers, Tom. 2001. *Anatomy Trains: Myofascial Meridians for Manual and Movement Therapists.* Philadelphia, PA: Churchill Livingstone.

Netter, F.H. 1997. *Atlas of Human Anatomy.* 2nd ed. East Hanover, NJ: Novartis.

Platzer, W. 2004. *Color Atlas and Textbook of Human Anatomy, Volume 1: Locomotor System.* 5th ed. New York: Thieme.

For conventional spellings of Sanskrit pronunciation, *Yoga Journal*'s online resource "Pose Finder," http://www.yogajournal.com/poses/finder/browse_categories.

For scholarly translations of Sanskrit terms, *The Cologne Digital Sanskrit Lexicon,* http:www.sanskrit-lexicon.uni-koeln.de/.

RESOURCES

The Breathing Project, Inc.—Educational nonprofit organization led by Leslie Kaminoff and Amy Matthews, providing advanced studies for movement educators and therapeutic classes to the public, New York, NY: www.breathingproject.org

Leslie Kaminoff's Yoga Anatomy website—The author's website, containing biographical and contact information, international teaching schedule, booking information, online training information, and his eSutra blog and other writing projects: www.yogaanatomy.org

Amy Matthews' Embodied Asana website—The author's website, containing biographical and contact information and full teaching schedule: www.embodiedasana.com

Krishnamacharya Yoga Mandiram—The yoga of T. Krishnamacharya and his teachings, founded by T.K.V. Desikachar, Chennai, India: www.kym.org

Bonnie Bainbridge Cohen's School for Body–Mind Centering—Embodied anatomy, developmentally-based movement reeducation and hands-on repatterning, El Sobrante, CA: www.bodymindcentering.com

Gil Hedley's Somanautics Human Dissection Intensives and DVD series—Workshops taught internationally: www.somanautics.com

Tom Myers' Anatomy Trains and Kinesis Myofascial Integration—Workshops and trainings taught internationally: www.anatomytrains.com

Ron Pisaturo—An actor, a writer, and a philosopher in the tradition of Aristotle and Ayn Rand: www.ronpisaturo.com

ASANA INDEXES
IN SANSKRIT AND ENGLISH

SANSKRIT INDEX

ARM SUPPORT POSES

ENGLISH INDEX

STANDING POSES

PRONE POSES

ARM SUPPORT POSES

JOINT INDEX

Note: Asterisk (*) indicates art or textual reference only.

Joint		Page number
Spine	*Cervical spine*	27*
		100-102
		190-192
		199-200
		220-221
		232-233
		243-245
	Lumbar spine	27*
		82*
		93-95
		128-129
		150-152
		168-169
		204*
		226-227
		249-252
	Thoracic spine	27*
		147-148
		150-152
		201-202
		226-227
		232-233
		240-242
		247-248

MUSCLE INDEX

Note: Asterisk (*) indicates art or textual reference only.